PILATES
for better Sex
The Ultimate Pleasure Guide For Women

MICHELLE JERMY

Pilates for Better Sex
The Ultimate Pleasure Guide For Women

With so many individuals to thank; where to start? Let's start at the beginning. A special thank you to the women that attend my classes for those ladies I personally train on a regular basis. For everyone that supports me, remember the beginning? When we were running exercise sessions in cold village halls...

Fifty Shades of Grey unleashed me! We often bantered in class but it was my lovely members that embraced my quirky side and allowed me to be ME. We explored ideas and I researched more and more; the science behind Pilates and good sex is there, I had found my calling.

Friends and family nurtured me and watched me flourish. The Core Studio was born. I continued writing and whilst working with Sarah Swift (a local photographer) we had many fun photo sessions but our final photo session with Richard Taylor (Tiger Fitness) was amazing. He was truly professional. For someone with little modelling experience, the camera loved him and well the photos were perfect, the positions were great fun, tough job but someone had to do it!

The response I got when I shared my book idea was immense. I was overwhelmed with the beautiful messages from women globally showering me with their kind words and gratitude. Many thanking me for taking a taboo subject and putting it out there. I joined a local women's in business group and the ladies are diamonds, some really took the time to share ideas to support my book, Karen Faulkner-Dunkley, thank you, please keep enjoying those long walks in the country. At a National Conference I met Vishal Morjaria and started my journey with him. I know I wasn't easy but I promised to be worth it! Thank you Vishal for your patience and Naval Kumar I always felt you were there to offer support and guidance, much appreciated.

Now to my KSFL family; Rachel Holmes I love running an idea past you, you manage to break it down in seconds and throw out any reservations I may have. Helen Tite I'm looking forward to working with you, I know we will have some fun times whilst making many people happier and healthier, I'm ready to fly the freak flag.

Finally lets be honest I wrote the material, Sarah provided the photos but Garry has done a true work of art with the book design. Now I have worked with Garry for a number of years and he just gets me when I say 'can we make it a little more girly?'. I have to say the book looks professional, it is perfectly presented has enough femininity and sensuality to take it under the sheets, I m very pleased. I even had book angels; Rachel Ellis, Claire Dutton and Lauren Day, much love.

The few months leading up to the launch had been particularly stressful and for those that held me through, I will always remember.

© Michelle Jermy Fitness 2016

All rights reserved. No part of this publication may be reproduced, stored in a retrieval system, or transmitted in any way or by any means, electronic, mechanical, photocopying, recording or otherwise, without the prior written permission of the copyright holder.

Designer - Garry Howell
Photographer - Sarah Swift
Male Model - Richard Taylor

Publisher's note: The reader should not regard the recommendations, ideas and techniques expressed and described in this book as substitutes for the advice of a qualified medical practitioner or other qualified professional. Any use to which the recommendations, ideas and techniques are put is at the reader's sole discretion and risk.

Bonus Material
FREE 10 minute Pelvic Pleaser Home Workout.
FREE Passionate Pilates Home Workout.
FREE MJ Tips to Looking & Feeling a Goddess of Love.

Foreword

Dear Reader

I admire Michelle's innovative approach within health and fitness. She has taken a taboo subject and made it her own. She has a gift and is willing to share. Her personality will embrace you and allow you to securely open up; she teaches you that you do not have to be the youngest, slimmest or even prettiest. Confidence is a mindset; self-love comes from within. Michelle has shown you how to gain confidence and self esteem which transfers into the bedroom.

Michelle has much credibility in the industry. Pilates for Better Sex is a celebration of her work and intimate close working relationships over many years. You will desire more passion and enjoyment in your bedroom. Pilates for Better Sex is a book that you will enjoy reading.

Raymond Aaron
New York Times Best Selling Author

Pilates for Better Sex

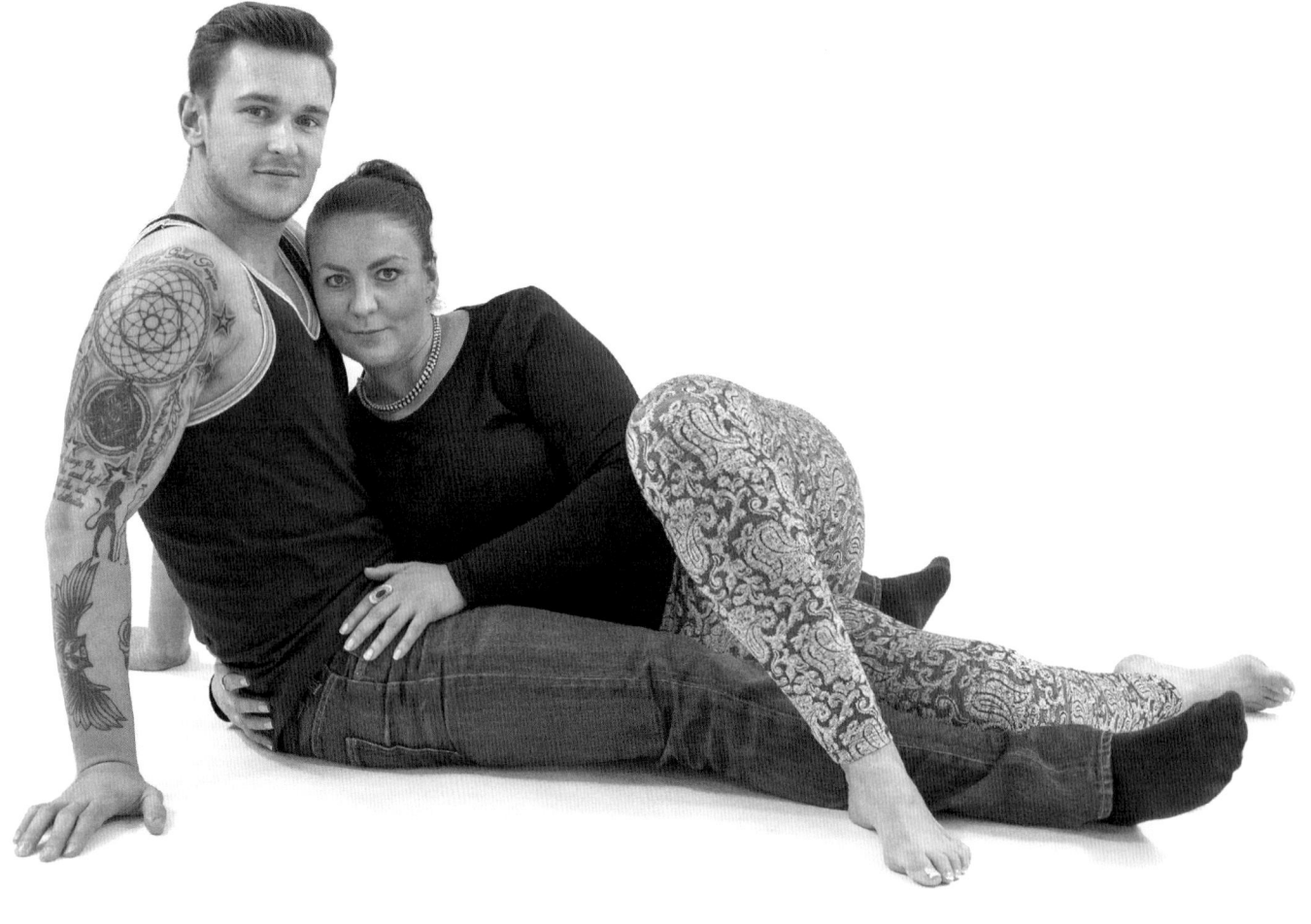

My Message to You

As women we often forget our own needs and put those of others before ourselves. In my experience this is also evident in the bedroom – many women do not enjoy loving sex, it is often seen as a chore. Sex releases so many feel good hormones, great sex is essential for optimal health, we need better sex! I smile as I write this, I have been on both ends of the sexual pleasure spectrum and when I realised my purpose, my gift; I had to share my secret to great sex.

For those yet to meet or know me, I take an innovative approach within health and fitness, I infuse personality, approach from different angles (excuse the pun) to inspire women to be the best version of themselves. I use Pilates, Nutrition and NLP, aiming to increase self-esteem and confidence.

Working as an exercise specialist for over 15 years I see the same pattern, many of my female clients experience low self-esteem and confidence, usually as a result of losing their identity due to motherhood, marriage/divorce, career/work pressures, we tend to put ourselves way down on the priority list. This directly impacts our personal relationships and with so many relationships not communicating effectively many need support to open up and allow themselves to discuss the 'real' issues, the issues so many steer away from. Regular Pilates, good nutrition and NLP has seen and continues to see so many women reach their goals and more importantly enjoy the journey. Positive lifestyle choices has a direct impact on their personal relationships, I receive many messages thanking me for supporting them on their journey and how they feel closer and more intimate with their partner; enjoying more love, more sex. Sounds good? Who wants more?

I was intrigued; this led me to research the theory behind Pilates for Better Sex. In the past, we didn't often see Pilates and Sex in the same sentence. An important part of any relationship is a healthy sex life and the basics of Pilates offers so much in making sex more pleasurable.

This book will take you through the science part of how Pilates tones the pelvic floor and more importantly how this relates to improving the sexual experience. There are over 50 Positions from Jermy (the new 50 Shades of Grey) you will be able to choose a number of exercises depending on your ability; Pilates poses and exercises including squats, pelvic bridges, crunches and many of the stretches that open the pelvis, boast circulation maximising blood flow, triggering nerve impulses to the pelvic floor. You will find stronger muscles resulting in the ability to hold your favourite positions for longer with increased sensitivity enhancing your sexual experience. For an extra 'O' you will also find tight lipped tips to feeling sexually confident, learn how to really turn the heat up and I'll show you the sexual positions guaranteed to reach orgasm. Now let's put the va va voom back in the bedroom.

Much love & lots of ooooooooooo

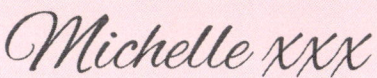

Contents

Chapter 1	The Secret, The Science Behind Sex	11
	• The Benefits of Pilates.	12
	• The Pilates Principles.	13
	• Pilates – The Core.	14
	• Pilates - The Pelvic Floor.	15
	• Let's Look At The Pelvic Floor.	15
	• Exercises & Devices To Strengthen The Pelvic Floor.	16
Chapter 2	Have Better Sex, Get In Shape, Feel Sexually Confident	17
	• Fascinating Flirty Facts - The How & Why Pilates Makes Sex So Good.	18
	• Tight Lipped Tips To Feel Sexually Confident.	20
	• The Sex Doctors Advice to Drive Him Wild For You.	22
	• Man Vs. Women Some Light Humour.	24
	• Ready For Better Sex Health Disclaimer.	26
	• Be The Best Version Of You.	26
Chapter 3	Lets Heat Things Up - Warm Up	27
	• Posture - Standing Upper Body.	28
	• Standing Lower Body.	32
	• Let It Flow.	35
	• On Your Back.	36
	• On All Fours.	39
	• Let It Flow.	42

Chapter 4	Moves to Increase Staying Power – Strength Exercises	43
•	Standing Exercises.	44
•	On All Fours.	50
•	Lying on Front.	54
•	Seated.	59
•	On Your Back.	61
•	Let It Flow.	65
Chapter 5	Increase Flexibility For Deeper Enjoyment	67
•	Standing.	68
•	On All Fours.	69
•	Seated.	73
•	Lying on Front.	74
•	On Your Back.	76
•	Let It Flow.	81
Chapter 6	Position of Pleasure	
•	Take It Slow – Time for Foreplay.	84
•	Mission To The Moon.	86
•	Booty from Behind.	88
•	The Rider.	90
•	Flamingo.	92
•	Side Lie Loving.	94

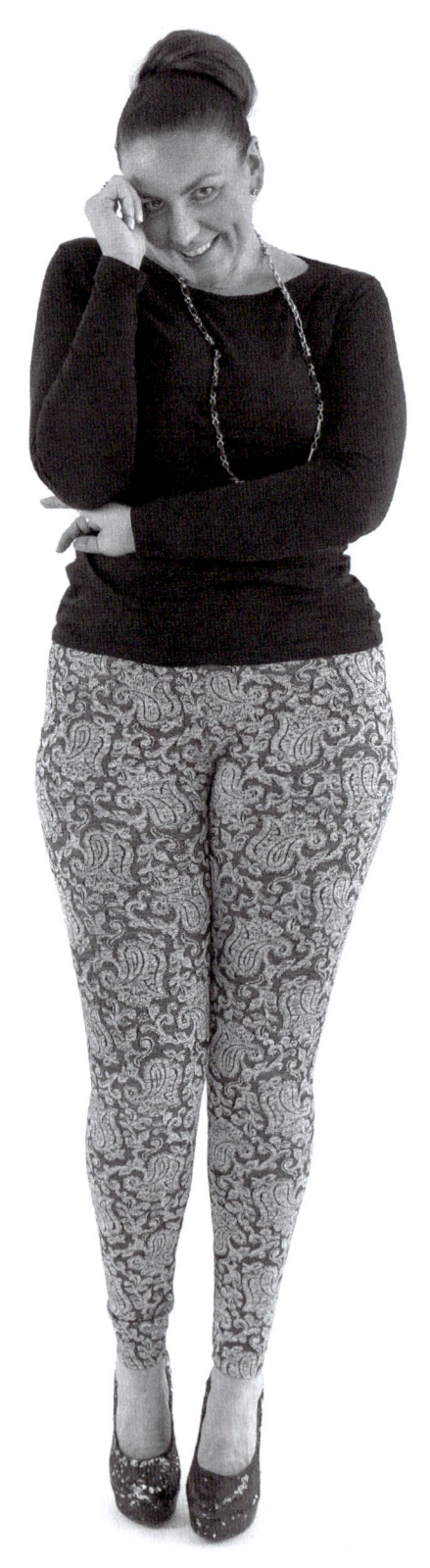

Chapter 1

The Secret, The Science Behind Sex...

Benefits of Pilates

Lets strip down Pilates for Better Sex, let the foreplay begin and explain the benefits of Pilates. The fundamental exercises start with the core of your body. When you strengthen and stabilise the core, you can safely move out from the centre. You can increase the movement of your spine, stretch your muscles and improve the range of motion in your joints. Using your breath, you refresh the body's cells. The heart pumps blood into your tissues and with training the deep muscles of your stomach, back and pelvis, you support your spine which provides stability in your pelvis and shoulders as you move.

In Pilates you will hear the term 'Pilates Principles' and you will learn to apply these principles to the Pilates movement. Exercises are performed as a whole mind and body experience and it is these skills that allow you to develop a deeper connection in the bedroom, helping you to bring your full attention to the movement. This enables the body to learn more from each exercise, leaving you yearning for more.

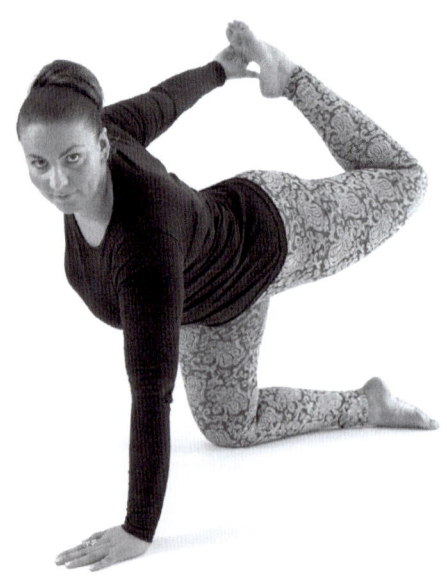

Pilates Principles

The Pilates Principles include: *Centring, Concentration, Control, Precision, Breath and Flow.*

Centering
Physically bringing the focus to the centre of the body, you may hear the term 'powerhouse'. Pilates exercises start from the centre.

Concentration
Focus and give your whole attention, committing to every exercise will maximise the feeling from each movement and enhance the benefit.

Control
Every Pilates exercise is done with complete muscular control. No body part is left to its own devices. You will slow things down allowing more control and perfect technique.

Precision
In Pilates, awareness is sustained throughout each controlled movement. There is an appropriate placement alignment relative to other body parts. You will focus on precision to perfect movement.

Breathing
Most Pilates exercises coordinate with the breathing, using the breath properly is an integral part of Pilates exercise.

Flow
Pilates exercises are performed in a flowing manner. Aim for fluidity, grace, and ease with all exercises.

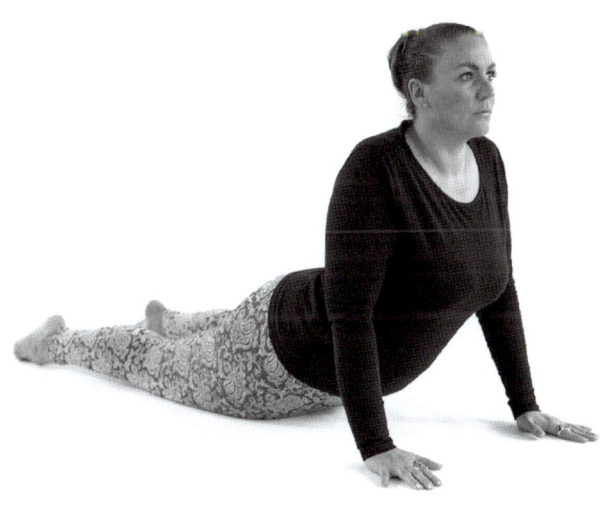

Pilates – The Core

There are a few basics related to how you use your core muscles - positioning of the pelvis and spine, and how to increase your range of motion that are used repeatedly in Pilates exercises. If you understand these moves, you will have a solid foundation in gaining maximum benefit from Pilates for Better Sex.

Pulling in the core (abdominals) is fundamental to the Pilates method of exercise. It is a technique that is promoted to some degree throughout the fitness world as a means of stabilising the spine.

When performed properly, you will create an integrated core of strength that supports the spine and provides stability and freedom of movement throughout the body. What is it to 'pull in the abs', 'engage the core', effectively?

In Pilates, we are looking to create a strong, stable position for movement. We develop this powerhouse or movement by employing the muscles of the pelvic floor and all of the core (abdominal) muscles, teaching them to work efficiently and in harmony with the muscles of the back.

Pilates puts a special emphasis on training the deeper abdominal muscles, such as the transversus abdominis. These muscles are often underdeveloped and not working equally with the often overworked surface muscles, such as the rectus abdominus (the six pack abs muscle).

Statements like 'pull your belly button to your spine', are often used to encourage a deep pull-in of the abs. These images, whilst they do convey the look of pulled in abs, can be misleading. They put the emphasis of the pull-in at the waist and may encourage a de-stabilising forward slump of the upper torso along with a tuck of the pelvis. The inner mechanics of creating a stable core begin not at the belly button, but with engaging the muscles of the honey pot; the pelvic floor.

Pilates – The Pelvic Floor (Honey Pot)

Working the pelvic floor muscles is not just for women bouncing back from pregnancy. The engagement of the muscles of the pelvic floor is critical to providing a stable base of movement. You feel like you are pulling the pelvic floor up and in toward the centre line. You might also imagine pulling the sit bones together. The only real difference is in intensity.

You might think my gym programme does not include any pelvic floor? Although I have just outlined to engage the core, the pelvic floor is the hidden treasure. So in the past pelvic floor strengthening may not of been high on the priority list but let's now put it there. A stronger pelvic floor will boost your core strength and stability, help reduce your risk of incontinence and for the purpose of this book improve your sexual relationships – yes you will improve your ability to reach orgasm.

So what, exactly, is your pelvic floor? Basically, it consists of the muscles, ligaments, tissues, and nerves that you never really think about, but actually really need. The pelvic floor acts like a hammock that supports your bladder, uterus, vagina, and rectum. So when the pelvic floor is weak, all of these areas cannot function as well as they should.

Let's Look At The Pelvic Floor

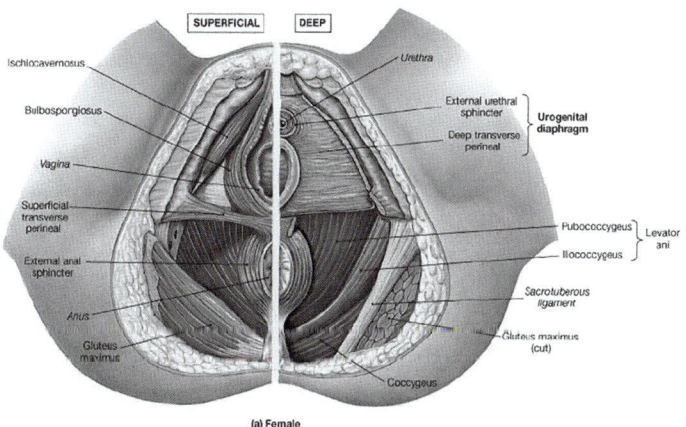

Diagram to show the Pelvic Floor. Here you can see the muscles, ligaments and tissues. Supporting your bladder, uterus, vagina, and rectum the negative consequences of weak or dysfunctional pelvic floor can lead to significant health complications affecting quality of life, which usually leads to confidence issues. Unfortunately many women feel uncomfortable to discuss pelvic floor and do not share their concerns.

This taboo subject needs to be brought to the forefront, we need to openly discuss and support each other.

Exercises & Devices To Strengthen The Pelvic Floor.

Pilates is an excellent exercise for strengthening the pelvic floor. In Pilates, for many of the moves the pelvic floor muscles are used to support. There is a firm and sustained engagement of the muscles where one is pulling the pelvic floor in and up, as part of the exercise.

The degree of engagement you use should be balanced with the amount of exertion you need to perform the Pilates exercise - hence why you will start at different levels. With Pilates for Better Sex, choose the exercises that are the right level for you. Some exercises might require just the slightest activation whereas an intense exercise will require a lot more from the pelvic floor and core (abdominals).

In addition to Pilates, please see below on how to do pelvic floor exercises anywhere! Visit www.pilatesforbettersex.com for further details and a review of a number of pelvic floor strengthening products currently available.

How to do pelvic floor exercises:

- *Close up your back passage as if you are trying to prevent a bowel movement and/or passing wind.*

- *At the same time, draw in your vagina as if you are gripping a tampon, and your urethra as if to stop the flow of urine.*

- *At first, do this exercise quickly, tightening and releasing the muscles immediately, up to ten times.*

- *Then perform slowly, holding the contractions for as long as you can before you relax: count up to ten seconds and repeat up to ten times.*

- *Look to complete two-three sets of ten every day: to help you remember, you could do a set at each meal or while waiting at the traffic lights during a car journey.*

Do remember to breathe throughout the movement and watch for the booty lift. You should not be clenching your booty. If you find it difficult to close both the front and back passage together without clenching your buttocks, then break it down and hold for less time. Do not be afraid to ask for help, we need to be comfortable to talk about the pelvic floor. Trust me, we all have the same concerns and fears.

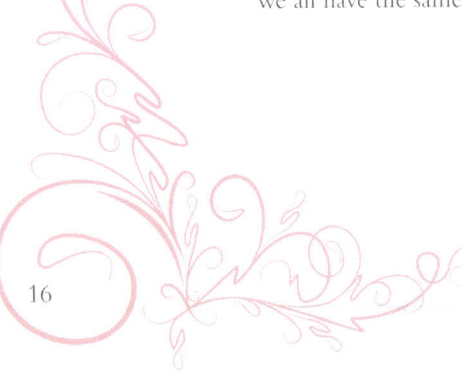

Chapter 2

Have Better Sex, Get In Shape, Feel Sexually Confident

**Fascinating Flirty Facts -
The How & Why Pilates Makes Sex So Good.**

Pilates for Better Sex is no different than Pilates for anything else. We do not do special Pilates exercises, well we may add a little extra spice.... Pilates is a full-body health and fitness workout and is going to be the foundation of a good sex life. Also Pilates gives you a longer, leaner, firmer body, you will feel and look sexier.

Fact 1 - Pilates increases physical stamina.
A key element to Pilates is muscle control. Joseph H. Pilates originally called his form of exercise "contrology". Control is the focus rather than speed. Less speed, think technique; as this is what produces results. Pilates gives you steady strength and stamina, transfer this is the bedroom and you will enjoy a longer, more intimate experience.

Fact 2 - Your body is your exercise equipment.
Unlike working out with machines at the gym, Pilates you are using your own body weight to perform the exercises. This is especially true with Pilates mat work, which was the original method of Joseph H. Pilates. Because sexual activity often requires you to use and sometimes support your own body weight, you will be able to enjoy yourself without any physical discomfort and will stay stronger for longer.

Fact 3 – Pilates teaches you to be fully present.

We are all familiar with how being fully present or "in the moment" enhances our life experiences. This is especially true during sex. One of the first things you learn with Pilates is focus and concentration. In order to work your body correctly, safely, and efficiently, you must concentrate throughout the exercises. You cannot be thinking about your to do list during sex; you must be fully present. Pilates trains your body and mind to be totally present. This will carry into the bedroom, enabling your to be totally present with your partner for a more intimate and enjoyable experience.

Fact 4 – Greater flexibility means more creativity.

Pilates gives you more muscle flexibility and improves the health of your joints. This allows you to get into positions you previously thought to be impossible. It also increases back and hip mobility, eliminating the back pain and restriction some women experience during sex.

Fact 5 – Increase blood flow equals more intense orgasms.

Pilates focus on "scooping" or pulling the "navel to the spine" which increases blood flow to the pelvic area. This continuous rush of fresh blood and oxygen to the sexual organs results in an increase in libido and more intense orgasms.

Fact 6 – Pilates reduces your stress level.

Stress is a significant reason couples have less sex. The Pilates method of breathing teaches you breath control. It was designed to cleanse the bloodstream through oxygenation, by bringing fresh blood to all of the cells. This method of breathing not only increases your physical health, it also reduces your blood pressure and triggers a relaxation response in the brain. Less stress equals more sex.

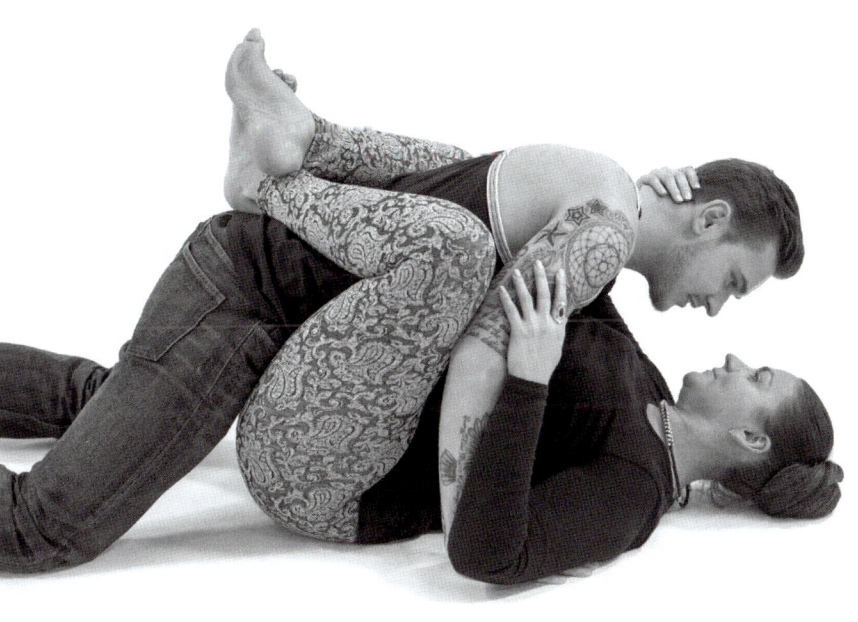

Tight Lipped Tips To Feel Sexually Confident

When you feel attractive you are less inhibited.

When you are physically fit and toned it gives you more self-confidence. Hesitation in sex has a lot to do with body image. You cannot have great sex if you are self-conscious about your body. Pilates teaches you to love your body and appreciate its unique strength, beauty and power. This allows you to be less worried about body image and have more fun. This benefit along with increased overall muscle strength, greater flexibility, healthy joints and greater self-confidence means that Pilates contributes to a great sex life well into your golden years!

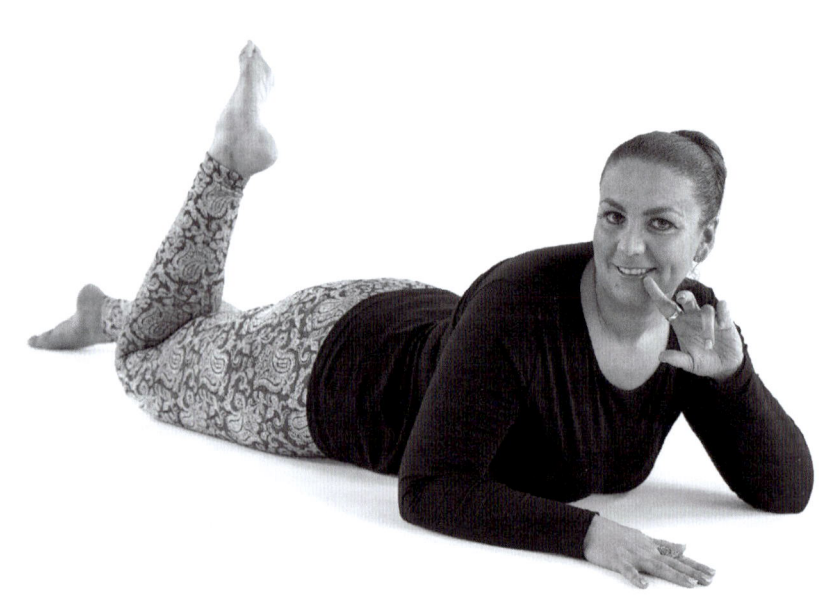

Tip 1 - Spend some 'me' time.
It may only be 10 – 30 minutes, ideas include; a hot bubbly bath with candles, listen to music, maybe a gym session or a walk in the countryside. Write down some of your favourite activities that ensure you fill yourself up. When we feel happy, we shine, we smile, we become more sexually attractive.

Tip 2 - Power of touch.
When was the last time or have you ever simply touched yourself? I mean take time to stroke your body, see what response it revokes. Enjoy, learn where you are most sensitive and take your time to enjoy the sensation, learn more about yourself. Obviously the ultimate power is to touch our honey pots. Masturbation is acceptable and can be wonderful to increase your arousal, release stress and make you feel highly sexual.

Tip 3 - Dress to Impress Yourself.
Now listen, remove your initial thoughts to dress to impress yourself. many women straight away think about dressing to impress their man. I want you to dress to impress yourself. This may mean, wearing heels, wearing a dress BUT it may also mean, a new hairstyle, new lipstick, new perfume or wearing matching underwear, what makes you feel gorgeous?

Tip 4 – Take a Slow Dance
We all have a number of songs that bring back many positive memories. Have you a song that you often think I would so love to get passionate to?
Listen to music that releases sexual feelings, allow your body to move, learn to enjoy the music and dance between the sheets.

Tip 5 – Read Something Raunchy
Us women have powerful minds. Use it positively - pick up a steamy, raunchy book and let your mind wander.

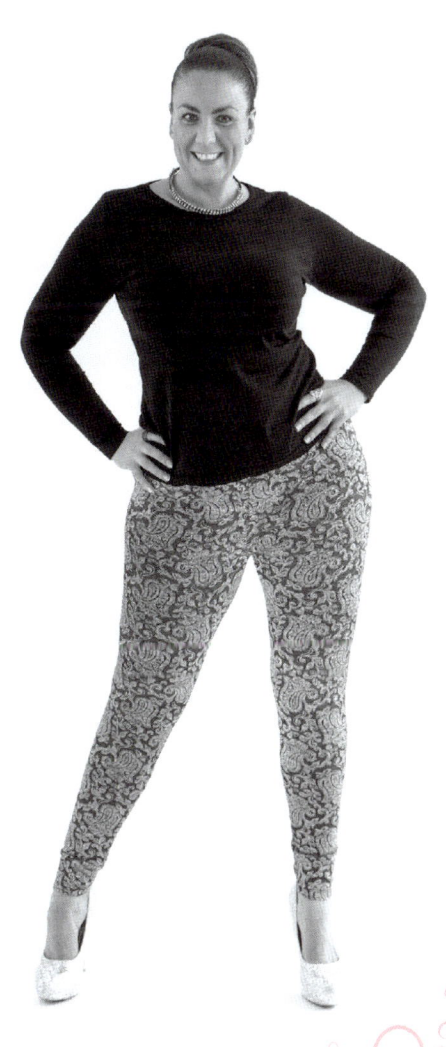

The Sex Doctors Advice to Drive Him Wild For You.

1. Date Night
Ensure you put aside time for each other. No children, no work, no technology. Yes I said it, all electrical appliances to be switched off & bye bye social media for one night.

2. The Power of Scent
Have you ever had a smell that brings back wonderful memories? Scent is so powerful. Maybe you recall the first perfume or aftershave you brought for each other?

3. Wear Something Raunchy
Maybe purchase a good fitting or uplifting bra. Or wear a shirt, top or dress with a little sweetness showing. Take your time to unbutton your shirt, top or dress - seduce him.

4. Touch Each Other
Touch without sex. Massage, stroke, kiss, caress and where possible look him in the eye.

5. Kiss for Longer
Kiss for a longer, slower, softer, sensual kiss. Stop to look at him, gently hold his head, stroke his hair. Increase your awareness to the body's response to the kiss alone, its magical.

6. Lie in Bed Naked
Allow your bodies to gravitate towards one another, the closer you grow, the more your bodies will connect physically and mentally. Lying naked with ensure skin to skin contact often and increases the intimacy.

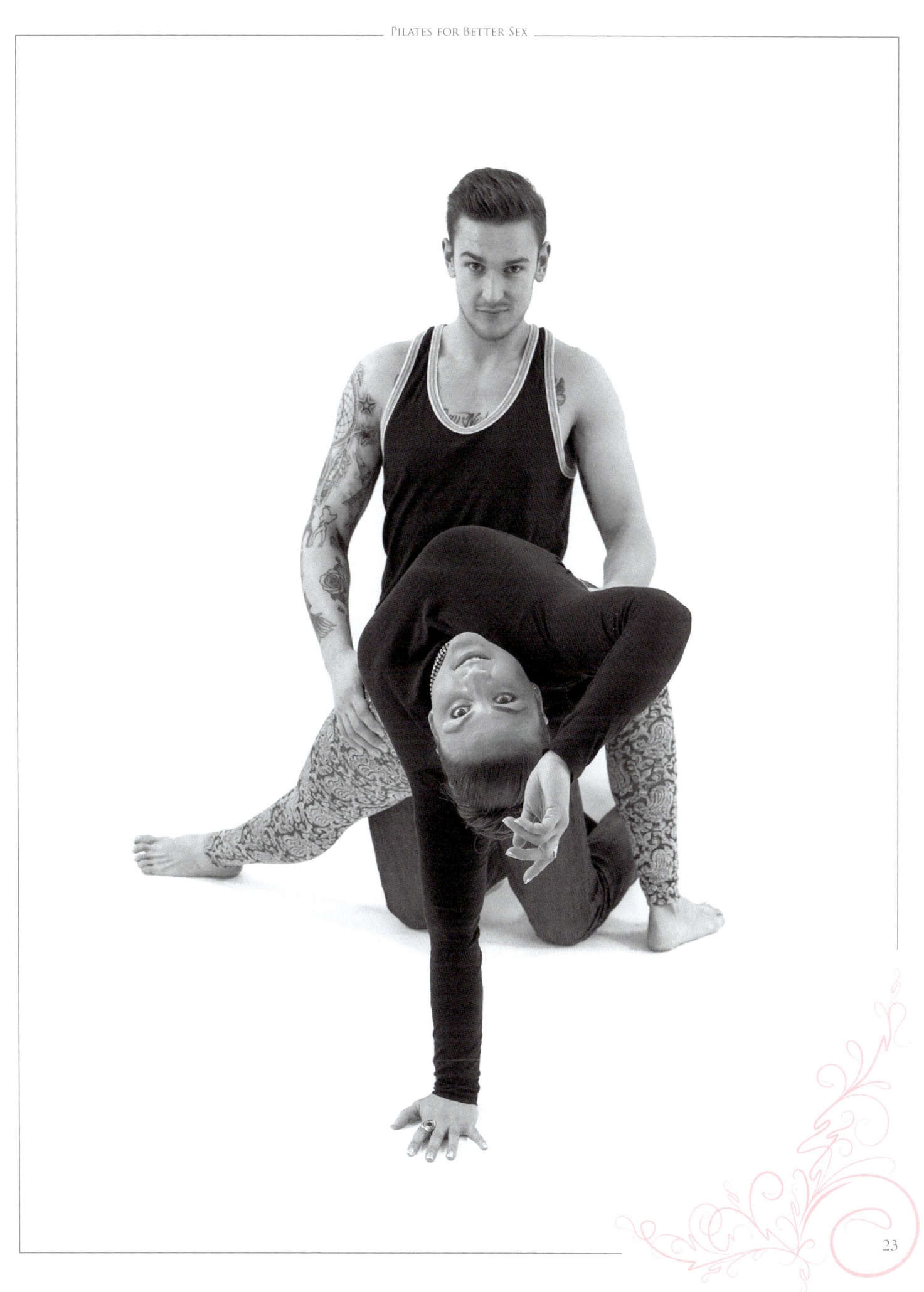

Man Vs. Women – Light Humour

Many of us will know the famous book Men Are From Mars, Women Are From Venus by Doctor John Gray. This story below outlines perfectly our differences. I want you to take the tips from above and just ride with them. Do not over think, do not question, just go. Trust me, men are far more simplistic in their needs and desires. We often have our preconceptions on what they think of us in the bedroom BUT it has been proven we are wrong. They do not see what we see, stop the self-destruct and increase the self-love. For my self-love presentations, workshops and courses please
visit www.pilatesforbettersex.com.

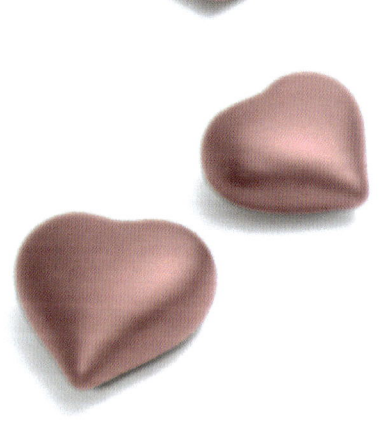
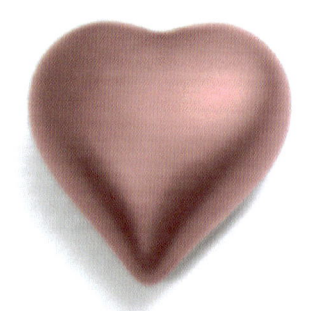

The story goes...

A store has just opened in Central London offering free husbands. When women go to choose a husband, they have to follow the instructions at the entrance:

"You may visit this store ONLY ONCE! There are six floors to choose from. You may choose any item from a particular floor, or may choose to go up to the next floor, but you CANNOT go back down except to exit the building!

So, a woman goes to the store to find a husband. On the 1st floor the sign on the door reads: Floor 1 - These men have jobs.

The 2nd floor sign reads: Floor 2 - These men have jobs and love kids.

The 3rd floor sign reads: Floor 3 - These men have jobs, love kids and are extremely good looking.

"Wow," she thinks, but feels compelled to keep going. Floor 4 - These men have jobs, love kids, are good looking and help with housework.

"Oh, mercy me!" she exclaims. "I can hardly stand it!" Still, she goes to the fifth floor and sign reads:

Floor 5 - These men have jobs, love kids, are gorgeous, help with housework and have a strong romantic streak.

She is so tempted to stay, but she goes to the 6th floor and the sign reads:

Floor 6 - You are visitor 71,456,012 to this floor. There are no men on this floor. This floor exists solely as proof that you are impossible to please.

Thank you for shopping at the Husband Store.

To avoid gender bias charges, the store's owner opened a Wife Store just across the street.

The 1st first floor has wives that love sex.

The 2nd floor has wives that love sex and have money.

The 3rd through 6th floors have never been visited.......

Ready For Better Sex – Health Disclaimer

There are many benefits associated with regular Pilates, though in order for the Pilates to be safe and effective, please consult with your doctor if you have a history of medical conditions and or injuries. Please note we all start somewhere and what was once your workout, will soon become your warm up.

Participating in the exercises from Pilates for Better Sex are at your own risk. If you are new to exercise, please ease yourself in and gradually build up. Ladies, if you are interested in heating things up in the bedroom, then this programme will be for you.

Please note: Risk of serious confidence and sexuality. Husbands may spoil you with gifts, boyfriends may propose. I take full responsibility for the positive side effects, with love.

Make today the start of something transformational. Embrace yourself, fall in love with yourself, believe you can and enjoy the journey to become the best version of yourself.

Body Confidence – comes from embracing the body you have.

Be the Best Version of You

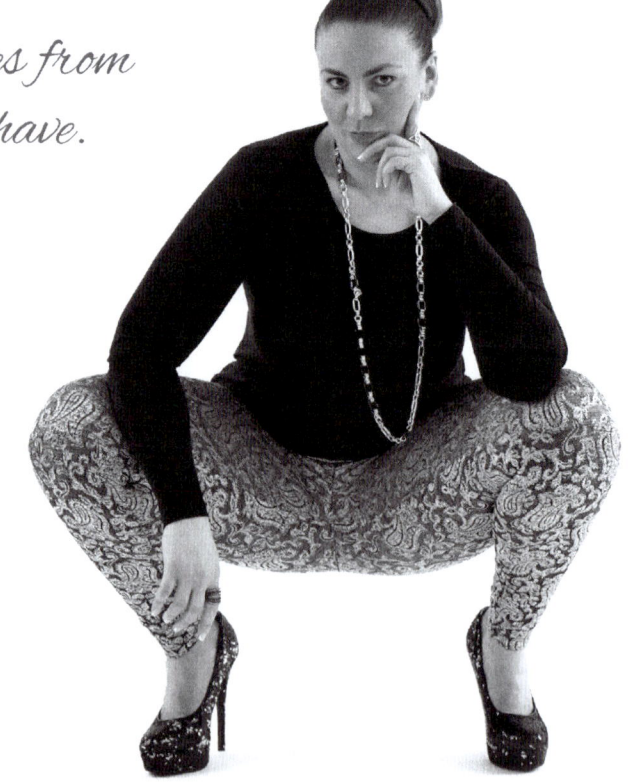

Chapter 3

Lets heat things up, warm up...

Standing – Posture

Pilates exercises combine strengthening with relaxation - they lighten the load on your spine and joints by correcting muscular imbalances, due to bad posture or misuse of muscles, alleviating tension. You will increase your mindfulness and awareness of your body. You will rediscover your body's natural movement patterns and this ability to tune into yourself, transfers to the bedroom and when you and your partner tune in together, magic happens.

When performing exercises, always strive to correct your alignment as this will directly impact the effectiveness of your workout. Use a mirror where possible to check your alignment and develop your ability to observe how your body moves. Also check your feet are in line with your knees and hips; your shoulders level and your waist long, lengthen through your spine. For floor exercises, use the mat as a guide. Work in the centre and keep the distances between the sides of the mat and your body equal during the workout. Truly take the time to check and respond to how the movement looks and feels.

Key Points for Standing Posture

- Hold the head centred at the top of the spine, lengthen through the body.
- Keep the shoulders even and relaxed.
- Be aware of how it feels to stand with the knees and ankles in line with the hips.
- Spread your weight evenly through the soles of the feet.
- Monitor your breathing, avoid the temptation to hold your breath.

Good posture reduces stress and strain on muscles and joints and ensures efficient breathing which results in more energy, better digestion, improved sleep, and increase well being.

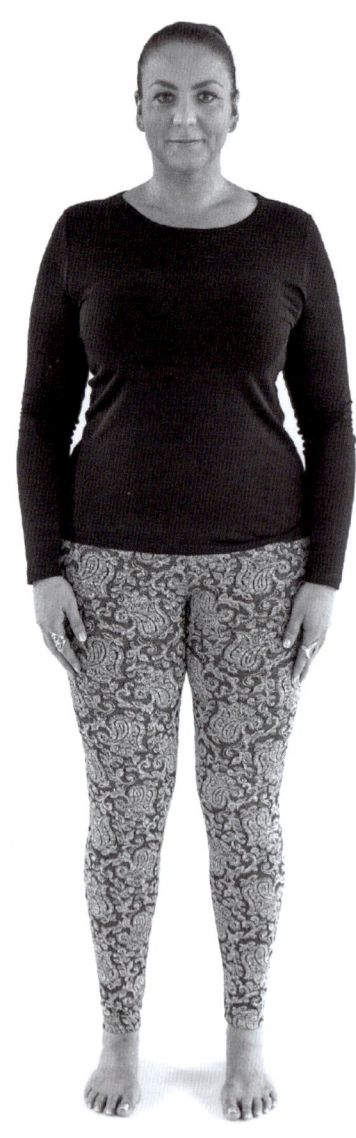

Standing Upper Body – Shoulder Movements

The shoulders are highly mobile but less stable than the hip joint as an example. It is important to warm the shoulders for those important hugs…..

Always maintain the key points for correct posture when performing standing exercises.

Purpose: To increase mobility/movement of the shoulders.

Bedroom Pleasure: HUG's, in all seriousness shoulder mobility is crucial for good posture and good posture leads to many benefits.

Repetitions: Repeat up to 8-12 times.

1. Stand with your weight evenly distributed and lengthen through the legs, spine and neck. Gently squeeze your booty and keep the belly button drawn in. Raise arms up to the ceiling and out to the sides, the arms make a 'V' shape.

2. Drawing your elbows down to your waist, imagine you have a grape between your shoulder blades. Retract the shoulder blades, opening the chest. Return to starting position and repeat.

Checkpoints

- *Do not lock the elbows.*
- *Lower only as far as you can control.*
- *Avoid tension through the neck.*
- *Breathe out as you pull the elbows into the waist.*

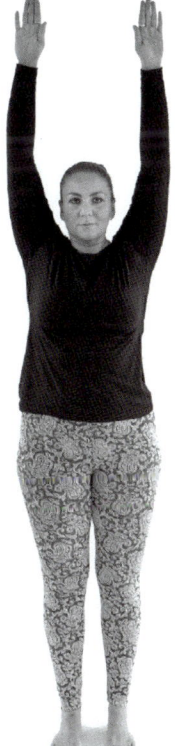
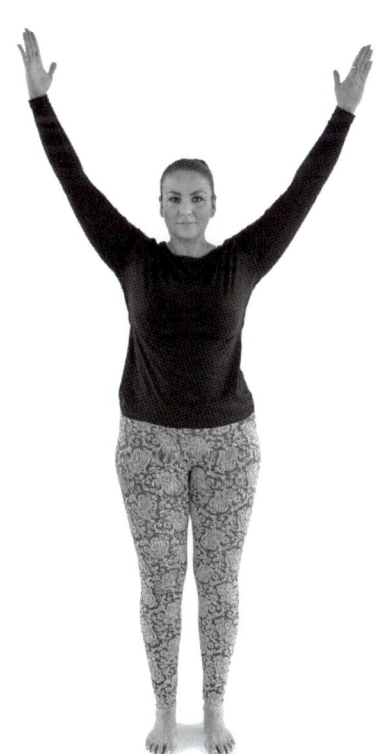
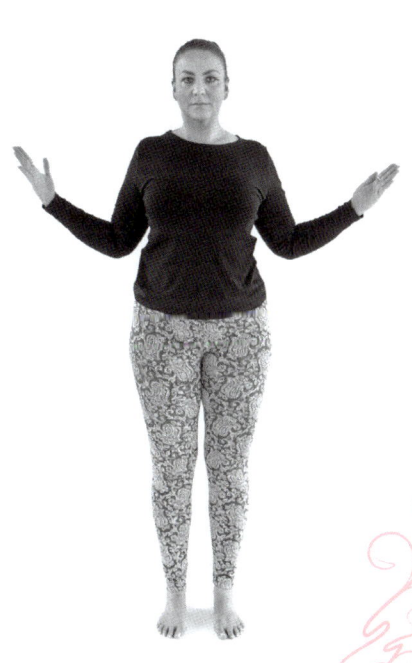

Upper Back Release

Modern lifestyle can result in tension. The upper back and neck hold the tension leading to headaches. Releasing stress can increase our willingness for bedroom activity. One of the common excuses for refusing sex……'I have a headache', though may I add sexual 'pleasure' has been proven to reduce headaches. This stretch releases the tension from the upper back and neck.

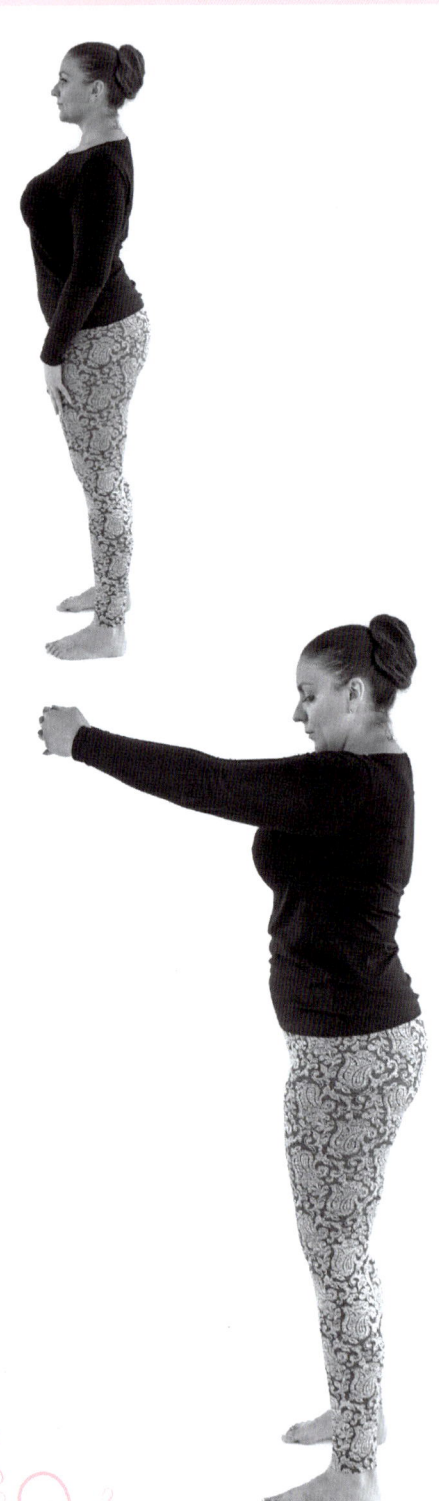

Always maintain the key points for correct posture when performing standing exercises.

Purpose: Release tension.

Bedroom Pleasure: Less stress, increased ability to focus on pleasure.

Repetitions: Hold the stretch for up to 10-15 seconds.

1. Stand with your weight evenly distributed and lengthen through the legs, spine and neck. Gently squeeze your booty, keep belly button drawn in.

2. Lift and extend both arms to chest height, gently drop chin towards chest and reach arms as far away from the body as you comfortably can, feeling a stretch across the upper back.

Share loving physical touch with those close to you, hug often, its beautiful!

Checkpoints

- *Do not create further tension through neck by lifting shoulders.*
- *Breathe throughout the stretch. Take slow deep breaths, clear your mind.*

Upper Body Opener – Chest Stretch

Through poor posture we can often find our shoulders become rounded and the chest becomes tight. The Upper Body Opener releases the chest. Now in the bedroom, the more we can draw the shoulders down and back, open and the lift the chest, the more our assets are on display and we have this confident radiance.

Always maintain the key points for correct posture when performing standing exercises.

Purpose: To open chest, improve posture.

Bedroom Pleasure: Own the bedroom when you walk in!

Repetitions: Hold the stretch for up to 10-15 seconds.

1. Stand with your weight evenly distributed and lengthen through the legs, spine and neck. Gently squeeze your booty, keep belly button drawn in.

2. Place your hands onto your booty, keeping shoulders down and back, squeeze your elbows towards each other until your feel the chest open.

3. Alternatively you can bring your hands behind your back, placing the palms together, retract the shoulders and hold. Please note shoulder mobility is needed for the alternative stretch, choose what is most comfortable for you.

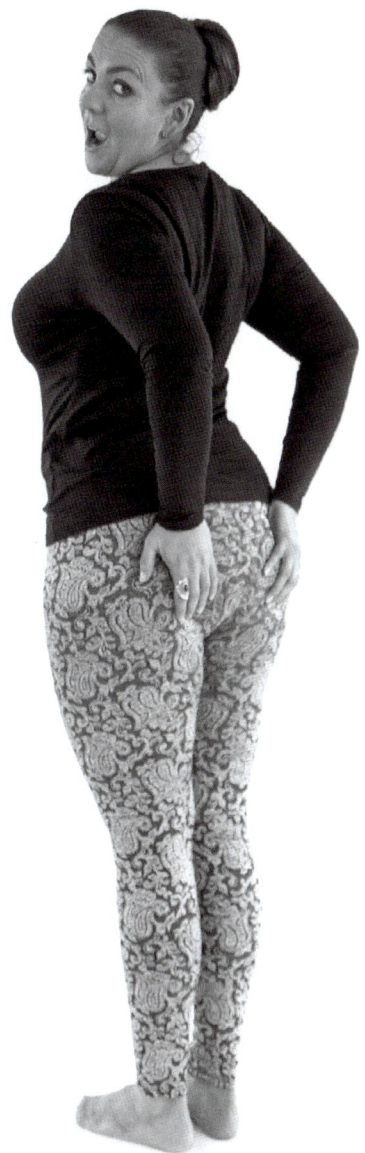

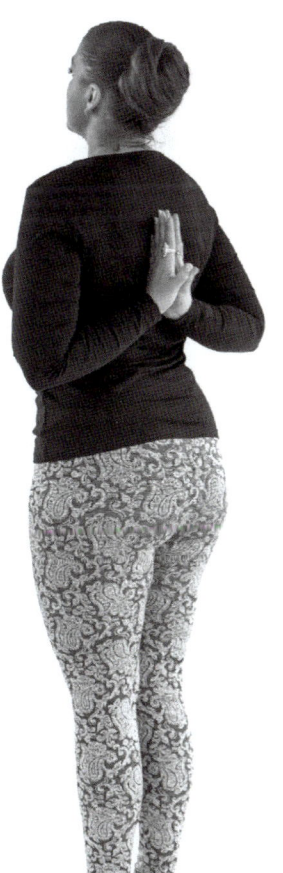

Checkpoints

- *Do not create further tension through the neck by lifting the shoulders.*
- *Breathe throughout the stretch. Take slow deep breaths, clear your mind.*

Standing Lower Body – Roll Down

This practices flowing movement and challenges the core muscles to control the spine. This teaches you to breathe with movement, relax into positions and respond to your body. As you perform the roll down, you will become aware of where you hold tension and when your body may resist certain movements or positions. Learn to let go and flow.

Purpose: Learn to flow and respond to your body.

Bedroom Pleasure: When you can respond to your body you transfer the skills to the bedroom.

Repetitions: Repeat up to 8-12 times.

1. Stand with your feet slightly apart in your natural stance. Your spine should be neutral, neither arched nor tucked under. Feel the movement coming from your core.

2. As you breathe out, scoop the tummy, nod the nose down, and peel the spine down to the floor: first the head, then the shoulders. Arms hanging loose, let the arms drop heavily towards the floor.

3. Roll the spine as far as you can without allowing the booty (tail bone) to rise up. Keep the pelvis upright. Breathe in. Then breathe out and gently peel back to standing position.

4. As an option, you can roll down half way and support your weight on your thighs, gently alternating a knee bend. Press the knee forward, lifting the heel and repeat on the other side.

Checkpoints

- *If you feel strain in your neck or shoulders, build the movement up slowly until you have released all tension. Learn to let go of any tension in your arms and neck completely.*

- *Soften through the knees if the back of your thighs are tight. Following the programme the flexibility in your thighs will improve significantly.*

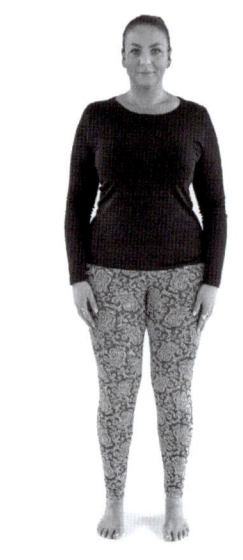
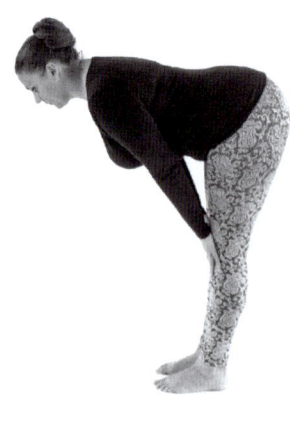
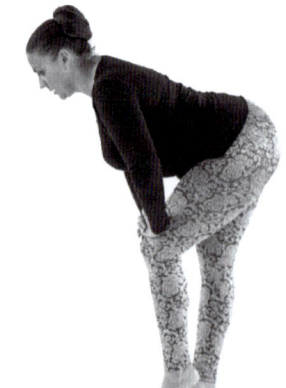

Hip Opener

The hip joint is renowned to be stiff, limiting movement and for many women hips and lower back can cause discomfort on movement. By gently introducing movement to the joint, it soon responds and over time you will start to notice more movement, greater strength and improved flexibility. Now considering many sexual positions need you to maintain positions whereby your legs are open, mobile hips with strong and flexible supporting muscles are essential to allow you to really get into positions with ease.

Always maintain the key points for correct posture when performing standing exercises.

Purpose: To increase mobility/movement of the hips.

Bedroom Pleasure: Hold sexual positions.

Repetitions: Repeat 8-12 times, each exercise.

1. Stand with your weight evenly distributed and lengthen through the legs, spine and neck. Gently squeeze your booty, keep the belly button drawn in.

2. Knee Lifts - Placing your weight onto one foot, lift the knee up to hip level, maintaining tall through the spine, control the movement hold for a second or two and gently place the foot back down, repeat on the other side.

3. Side to Side - The second exercise; keeping the weight on the opposite foot and maintaining neutral posture, take the leg across the midline as far as you can then out to the side, without coming out of neutral position. Repeat.

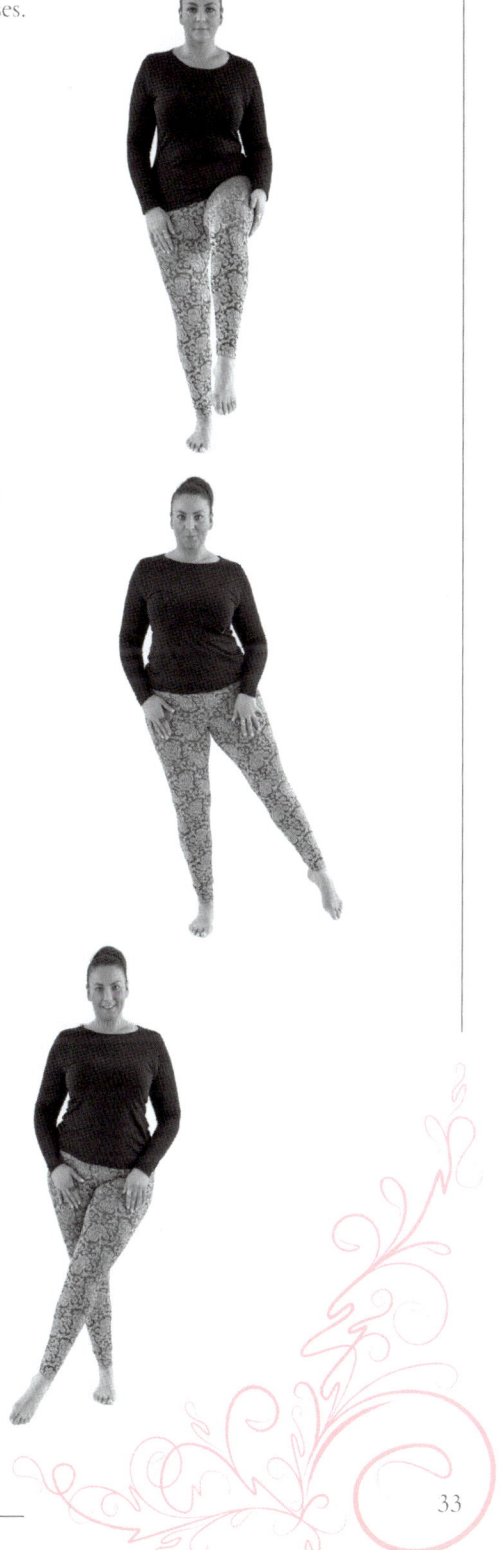

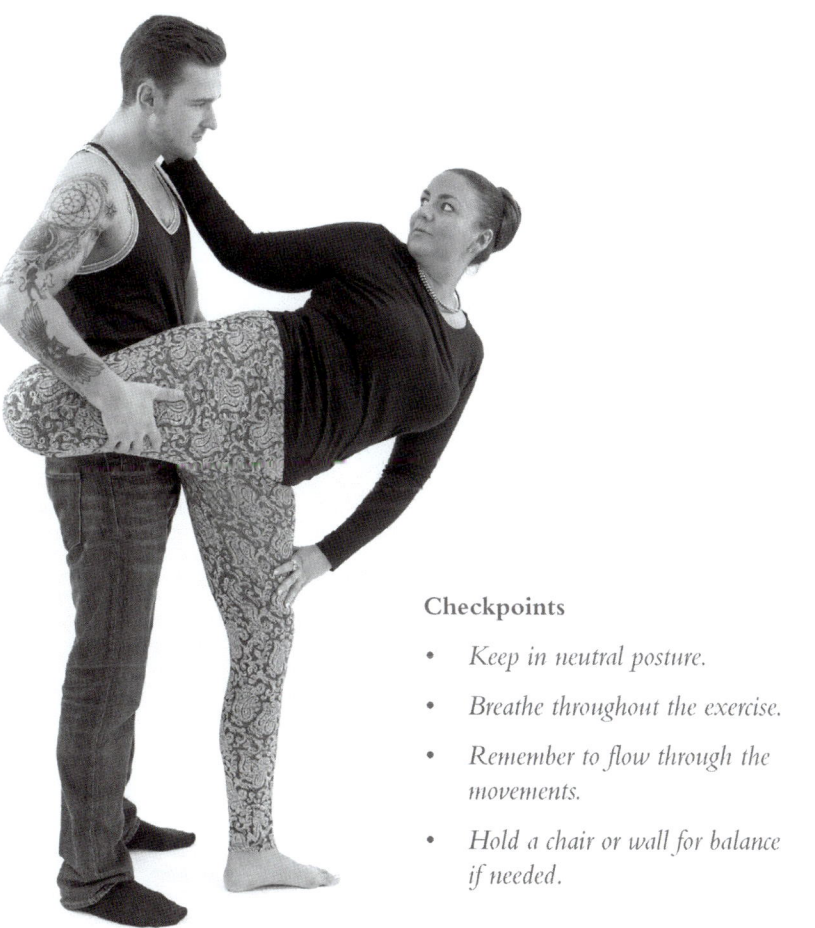

Checkpoints

- *Keep in neutral posture.*
- *Breathe throughout the exercise.*
- *Remember to flow through the movements.*
- *Hold a chair or wall for balance if needed.*

Back of Thigh Stretch

Lets go straight to the bedroom. Booty from Behind can be uncomfortable if you are tight on the back of the thighs. You are there, waiting to receive, ready for passion and at the point of excitement and ecstasy, you lean a little further forward and the tightness felt up the thighs consumes your thoughts. Your body goes tight, you can no longer relax and take the length, you were in the moment and now it's gone. The back of thigh stretch will resolve this.

Purpose: To increase flexibility of the back of thighs.

Bedroom Pleasure: Increase ability to hold positions when performing Booty from Behind.

Repetitions: Hold for up to 10-15 seconds, repeat 1-2 times.

1. Stand with your weight evenly distributed and lengthen through the legs, spine and neck. Gently squeeze your booty, keep the belly button drawn in.

2. Take a deep breathe in. As you breathe out, scoop the belly, nod the nose down, and peel the spine down to the floor: first the head, then the shoulders. Arms hang loose, let the arms drop heavily towards the floor and hold, ensure your breathe in and out whilst holding the position.

3. The legs can be hip width apart or practice in a straddle stance.

Checkpoints

- *If your hands cannot reach the floor, use a chair, bed or Pilates blocks to support your weight.*
- *Soften through the knees if you need.*
- *Remember the breathing, it is tempting to want to hold the breath.*

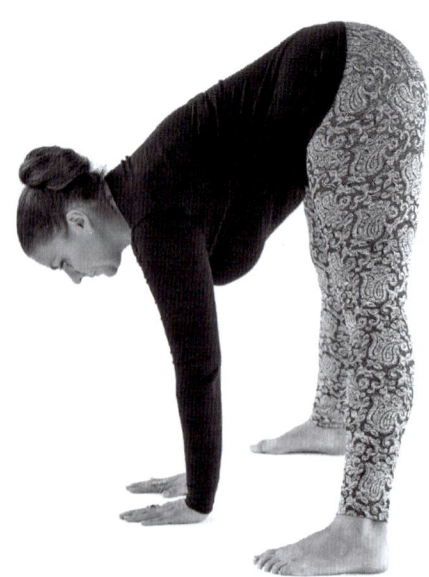
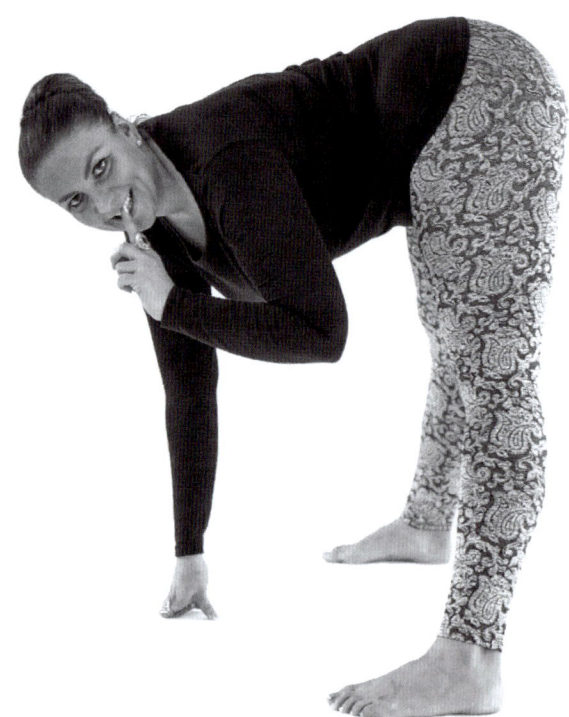

Let It Flow

Visit **www.pilatesforbettersex.com** for more ideas on routines for all levels.

Roll Down	32
Shoulder Movements	29
Upper Back Release	30
Upper Body Opener	31
Roll Down	32
Hip Opener	33
Back of Thigh Stretch	34

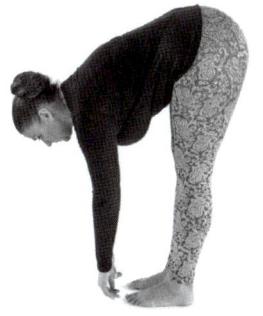
1

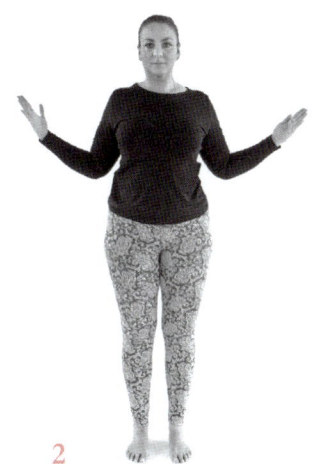
2

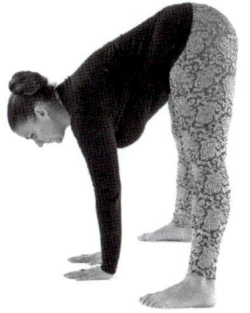
7

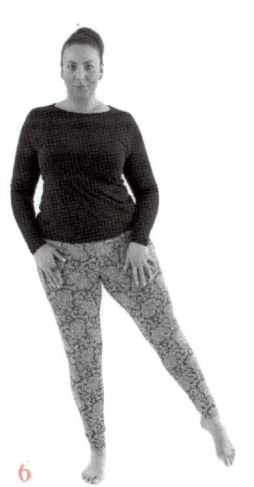
6

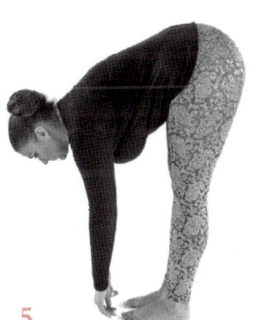
5

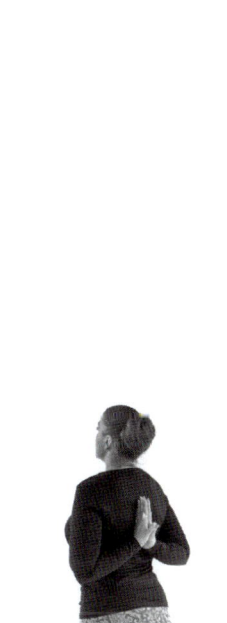
3

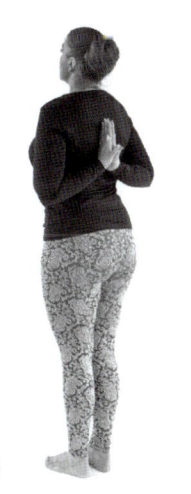
4

On Your Back - Pelvic Tilt Tease & Booty Bridge

This is a great mobiliser, will loosen a stiff back & increase blood flow to the pelvic area. The aim is for each bone in your spine to lift off the floor in succession. You may find that to begin with, your back lifts in two or three sections: try to create length between each vertebra. As you lower yourself, place each vertebra in turn on the floor.

The hips should be perfectly level, and you should try to create as much distance between your hips and your shoulders as possible. Do not forget to tilt the pelvis as you begin the movement. To mobilise the spine fully, be sure to return to neutral as you lower your back to the floor just before you tilt the pelvis and start the next tease.

Purpose: To mobilise the spine and challenge the core.

Bedroom Pleasure: Increase blood flow to the pelvic floor, increasing sensitivity and improving sexual pleasure.

Repetitions: Repeat 8-12 times.

1. Lie on your back with your arms by your sides, slide your shoulder blades down your spine and lengthen your arms away. Bend your knees and place your feet hip-width apart flat on the mat. Your head is in alignment and your spine in neutral.

2. Tilt your pelvis and lengthen the tailbone away. The whole length of your spine should be in contact with the floor.

3. Slowly peel your spine up off the floor bone by bone, raising your hips towards the ceiling and keeping the core engaged. Make the movement smooth and flowing.

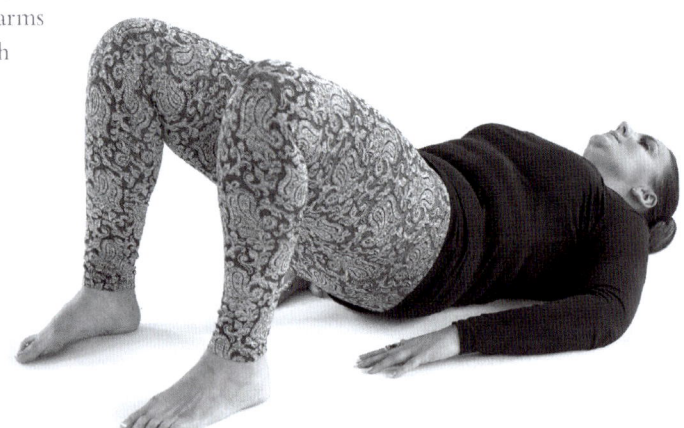

Pelvic Tease

Checkpoints

- *Keep the hips level.*
- *Maintain the distance between the hips and the ribs.*
- *Make the movement flow.*

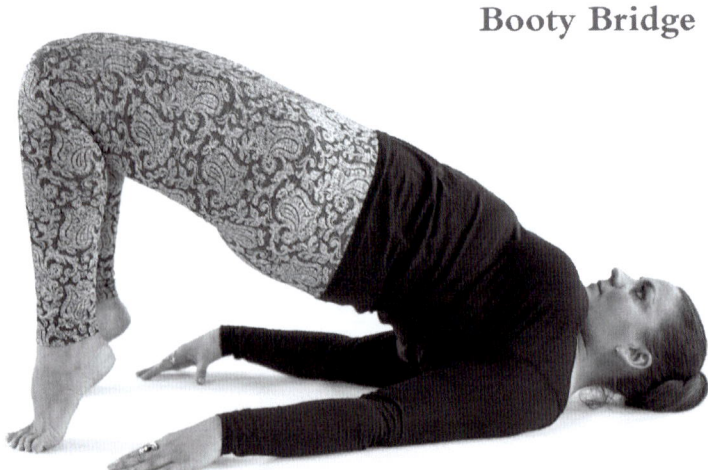

Booty Bridge

Curl & Hug

A great stretch for your back, releasing tightness. Give yourself time to tune into your body.

Purpose: To stretch and release your back.

Bedroom Pleasure: This position can transfer straight to the bedroom, let your partner slide in.

Repetitions: Hold for up to 10-15 seconds, repeat 1-2 times.

1. Lying on your back, bring your knees into your chest. Hold the knees gently, no direct pressure or hold at the back of you thighs.

2. For a deeper stretch reach and hold your heels, really add some resistance by hugging tight, curling through the body and then release.

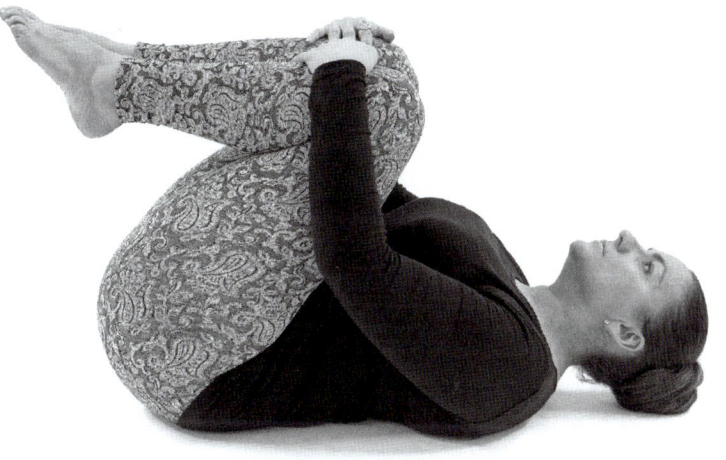

Checkpoints

- *Let the head and shoulders relax into the mat.*
- *Remember the breathing, it is tempting to want to hold the breath.*

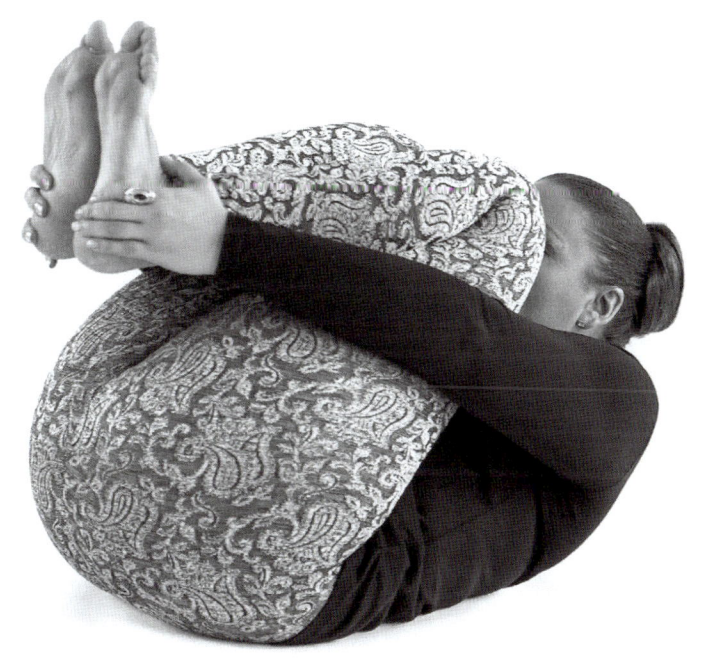

Full Body Lengthening

A great stretch for your whole body, release tightness and relax. Give yourself time to tune into your body and prepare.

Purpose: To stretch and release your whole body.

Bedroom Pleasure: Teaches you to truly relax and be in the moment.

Repetitions: Hold for up to 10-15 seconds, repeat 1-2 times.

1. Lying on your back, fully extend your arms over your head and lengthen through the legs.

Checkpoints

- *Let the head and shoulders relax into the mat.*
- *Remember the breathing, it is tempting to want to hold the breath.*
- *You can emphasise the extension on one side of the body before switching to the other side.*

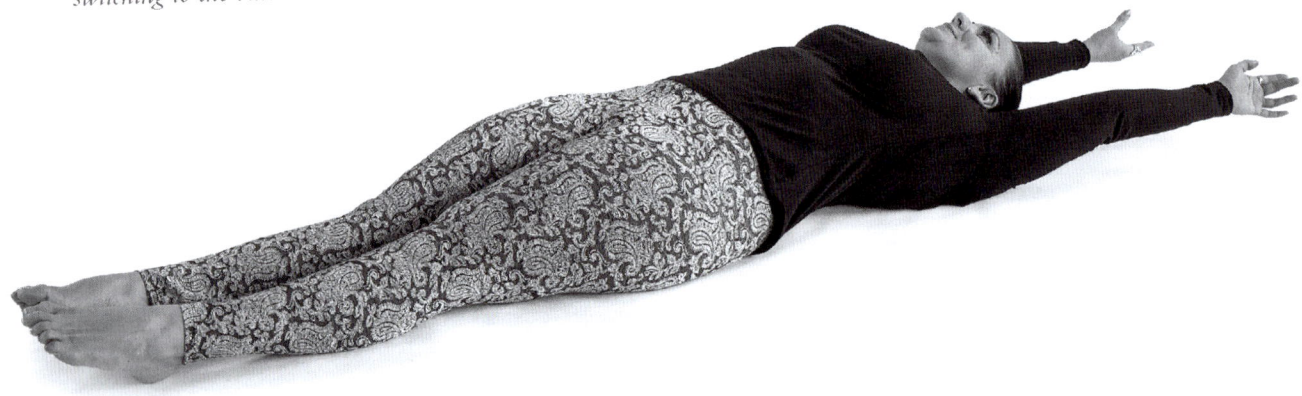

It's hard to feel beautiful when your thoughts are negative on your appearance. Keeping a positive mind is not only with regards to life but also on how you feel about yourself. Bring to light the things you love, if you struggle with this task ask those close to you.

All Fours – Curl & Release

Holding your body weight, to be able to move your hips with ease and feel confident, comes from the base exercise of the curl and release. This is a great starting point and over time you can progress to the strengthening exercises and/or stretches for deeper enjoyment.

Purpose: To increase movement through the spine and hips.

Bedroom Pleasure: Builds strength enabling more advanced sexual positions.

Repetitions: Repeat up to 8-12 times.

1. Kneeling on all fours. Consider the key teaching points for the all fours position. Bring your chin to your chest and tuck the hips under, curling up through the spine. You may prefer to rest on your knuckles opposed to palms to the floor.

2. Under control, tilt your tailbone to the ceiling, emphasising the booty whilst lifting the chest and looking forward.

Checkpoints

- *Use the breathing to increase the range of movement. Think about breathing out (exhale) on the effort.*
- *Ease through the movement, always remain under control.*

Key Points for on All Fours

- Position your hands under your shoulders and your knees under your hips.
- Spread your weight evenly. Pull the belly button in, gently tuck hips under and draw belly button in.
- Monitor your breathing, avoid the temptation to hold your breath.

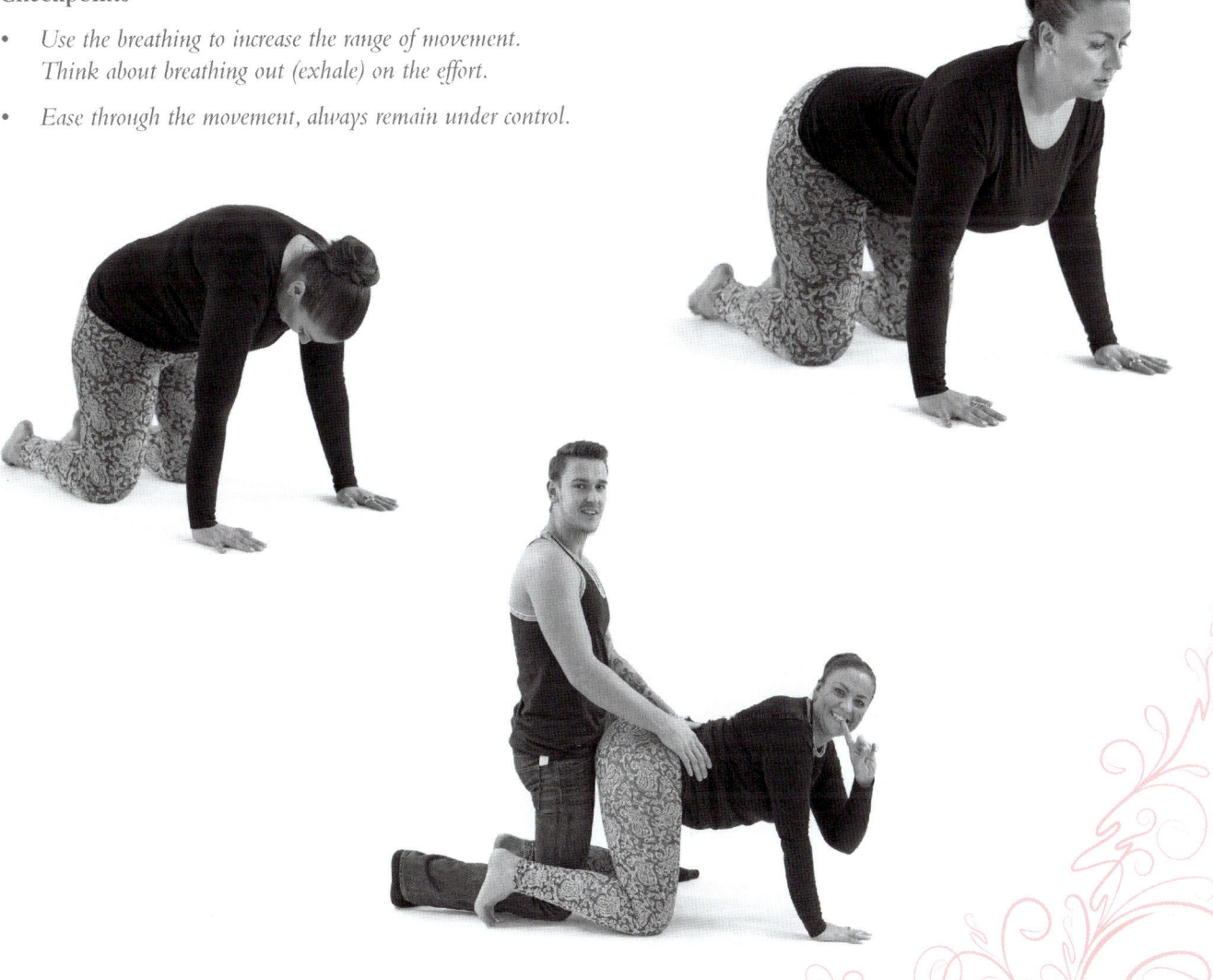

Sit Back & Hold

A great stretch for your lower back but also your shoulders, releasing tension and tightness. Give yourself time to tune into your body.

Purpose: To stretch and release your back and shoulders.

Bedroom Pleasure: This position can transfer straight to the bedroom, lift your booty slightly, let your partner slide in. Bring your arms back to support your weight and away you go.

Repetitions: Hold for up to 10-15 seconds, repeat 1-2 times.

1. Start in the all fours position. Push your weight back towards your heels, with your arms reaching out in front.

2. If you prefer sit with your knees wide, push you weight back and aim to bring your chest towards the floor.

3. Another option is to reach for your heels and pull into a small ball.

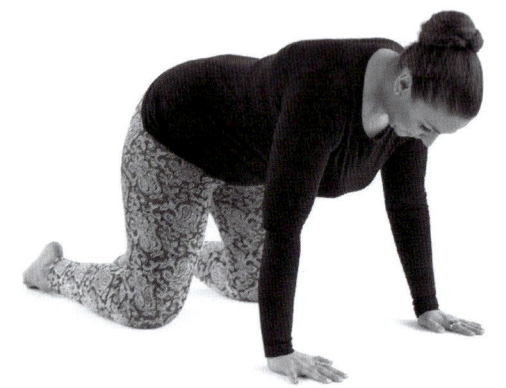

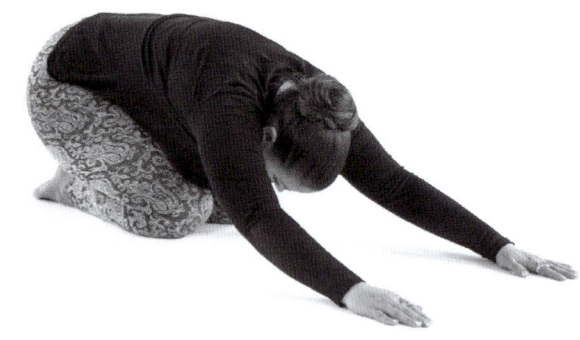

Focus on your best assets not the worst. Stop staring at the wrinkle or the bulge. Quit comparing yourself to the media representation of 'body beautiful'. Let your "worst" features recede and focus on your best instead. You have far more beautiful features than you see!

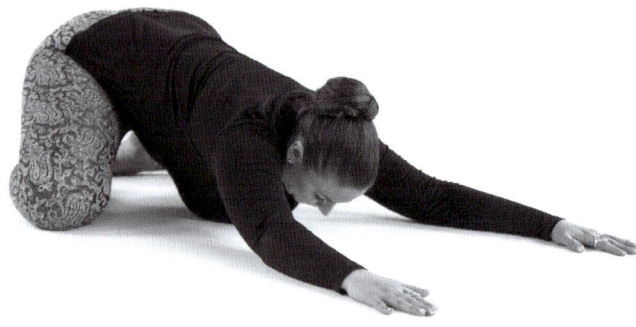

Checkpoints

- *Remember the breathing, it is tempting to want to hold the breath.*

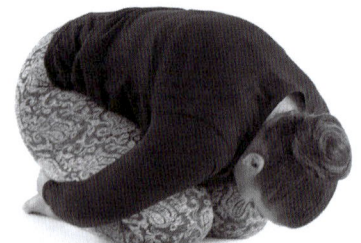

Bend Me Over

A great deep stretch for your lower back and back of thighs. This is more strenuous than many of the other stretches but once you can get into position, it feels great.

Purpose: To stretch and release your back and the back of thighs.

Bedroom Pleasure: This position can transfer straight to the bedroom, consider resting your arms on the bed to support your weight.

Repetitions: Hold for up to 10-15 seconds, repeat 1-2 times.

1 Start in the all fours position. Let your toes curl under, push through your hands, lifting your booty to the ceiling.

2 You are looking for a V shape, ankle, knee and hip in alignment, hip, shoulder, elbow and wrist.

3 Once in position, press your heels towards the floor and drive your chest towards your thighs, keeping the booty on show.

Checkpoints

- *Remember the breathing, it is tempting to want to hold the breath.*
- *If you need to soften through the knees take the option.*
- *The heels lifted will reduce the intensity of the stretch.*
- *Use a chair, bed or Pilates blocks to reduce the range of movement if new to Pilates or exercise.*

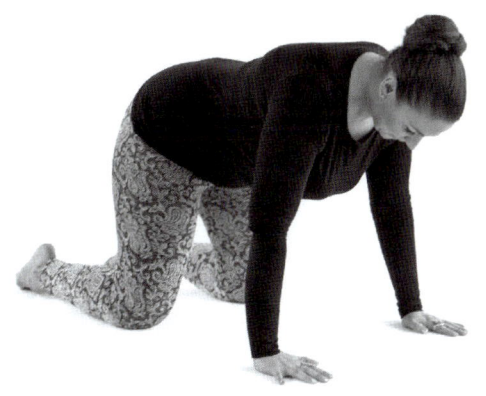

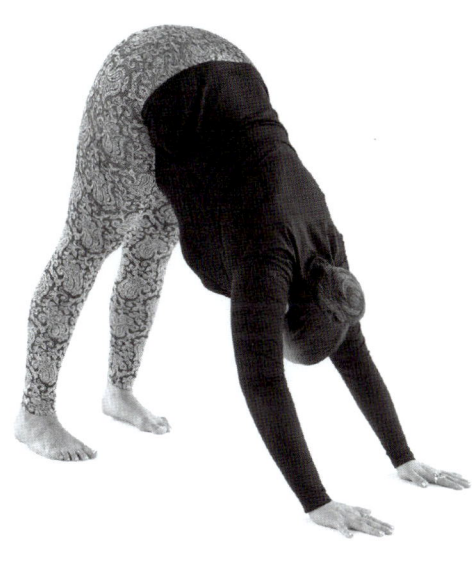

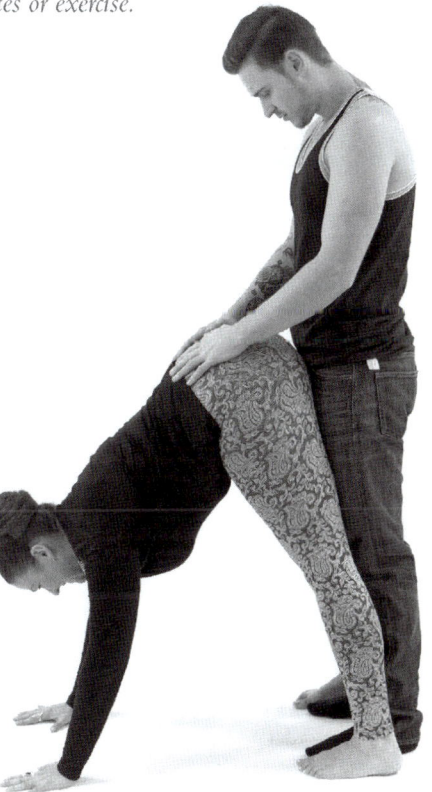

Let It Flow

Visit www.pilatesforbettersex.com for more ideas on routines for all levels.

Bend Me Over	41
Curl & Release	39
Sit Back & Hold	40
Full Body Lengthening	83
Curl And Hug	37
Booty Bridge	36

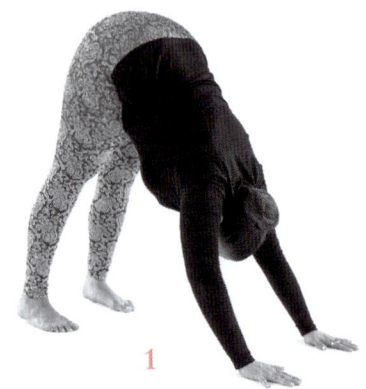
1

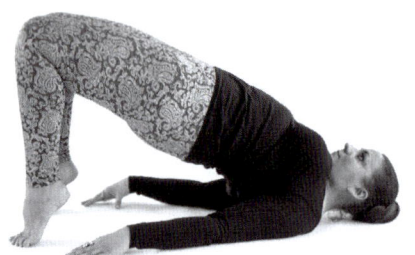
6

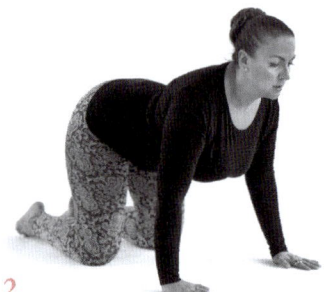
2

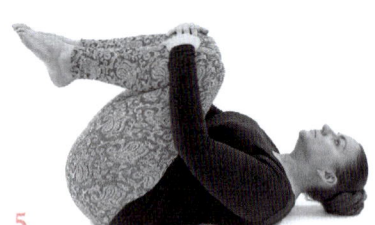
5

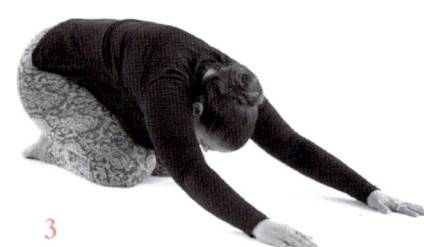
3

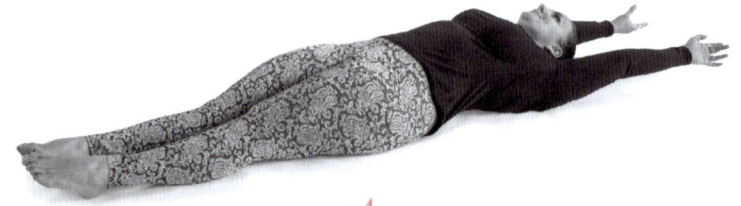
4

Chapter 4

Strength moves to increase staying power

Standing Upper Body - Arm Embrace

Always remember the key teaching points for posture when performing standing exercises. In the strength section, we take this warm up exercise and really focus on the draw down through the arms. Visualise squeezing a grape through your shoulder blades, encouraging the retraction of the shoulders, resulting in an increase in upper body strength and improved posture.

Purpose: To increase mobility and strength of upper body.

Bedroom Pleasure: Improved posture will mean you walk with more confidence.

Repetitions: Repeat up to 8-12 times.

1. Stand with your weight evenly distributed and lengthen through the legs, spine and neck. Gently squeeze your booty, keep the belly button drawn in. Raise arms up to the ceiling and take arms to the side (think of a V shape).

2. Drawing your elbows down to your waist, imagine you have a grape between your shoulder blades, retract shoulder blades opening chest. Return to the starting position and repeat.

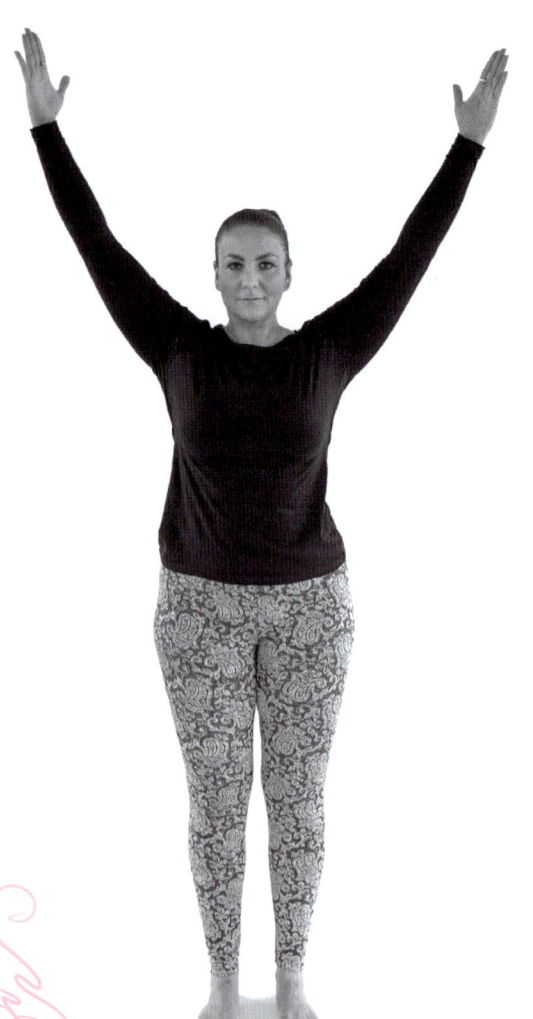

Checkpoints

- *Do not lock the elbows.*
- *Lower only as far as you can control.*
- *Avoid tension through the neck.*
- *Breathe out as you pull the elbows into the waist.*

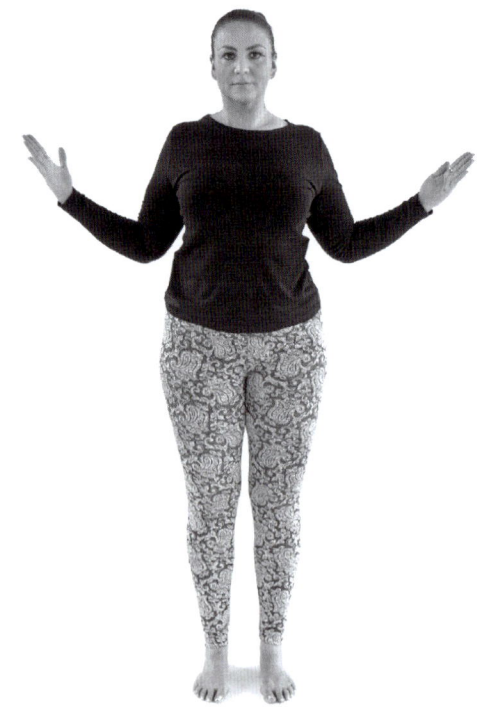

Standing Lower Body. - Wide Leg Press, Hold & Reach

Often I get asked what exercises to do for the booty, the pert bottom, firm and uplifted; full of desire. The exercise below focuses on the booty and thighs and works with legs apart, a familiar position for the bedroom.

Purpose: To increase strength of lower body and really firm the booty and thighs.

Bedroom Pleasure: As strong booty will open the opportunities to many advanced sexual positions.

Repetitions: Repeat up to 8-12 times.

1. Stand with your weight evenly distributed, then step feet as wide as you comfortably can with knees and toes pointing out to the sides.

2. Take a deep breath in and as you exhale, lower down as far as you can comfortably go. Do not let knees go over the toes.

3. Take a deep breath in as you breathe out push through your feet, squeeze through your booty and come back to standing.

4. As an option, you can lower down and pulse for four counts at the bottom before coming back to standing.

5. As in the photo, lift onto your heels as you return to standing, (on the extension).

6. Alternatively, when sitting into the position, hold and take the arms and reach above the head, over to one side, repeat on the other side then push out of the position and come to standing.

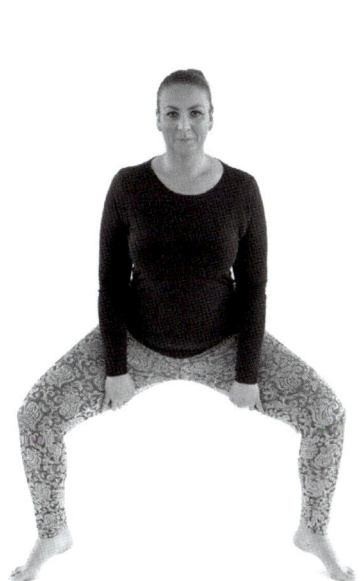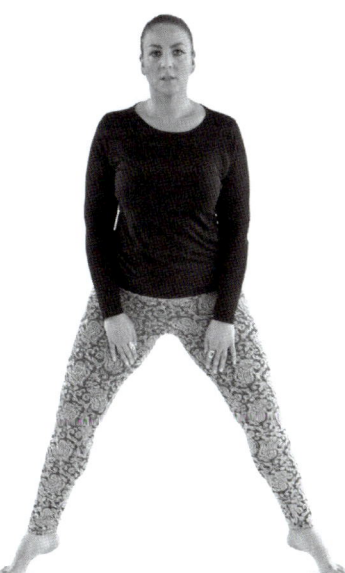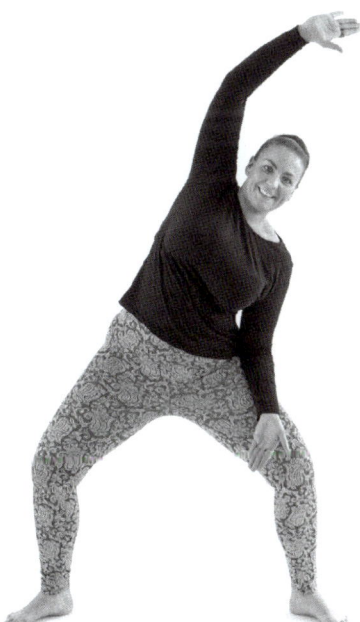

Checkpoints

- *Ensure knees and toes follow the same line.*
- *Lower only as far as you can control.*
- *Play with the options and see which ones really works for you.*

Tight Legged Squat

Staying on the booty theme. The Tight Legged Squat will build your stamina for holding positions. Once you are in a position, learning to breathe and staying relaxed is key. Enabling you to fully enjoy the sexual pleasure is a skill in its self.

Purpose: To increase strength of lower body and really firm the booty and thighs.

Bedroom Pleasure: A strong booty will open the opportunities to many advanced sexual positions.

Repetitions: Perform for 10-30 seconds, 1-2 sets.

1. Stand with your weight evenly distributed, then step feet together.
2. Take a deep breath in and as you exhale, sit your weight back, chest lifted and go down as far as you can comfortably go. Do not let knees go over toes. Hold these position.

Checkpoints

- *Ensure knees do not go over toes.*
- *Lower only as far as you can control.*
- *Ensure you breathe throughout.*

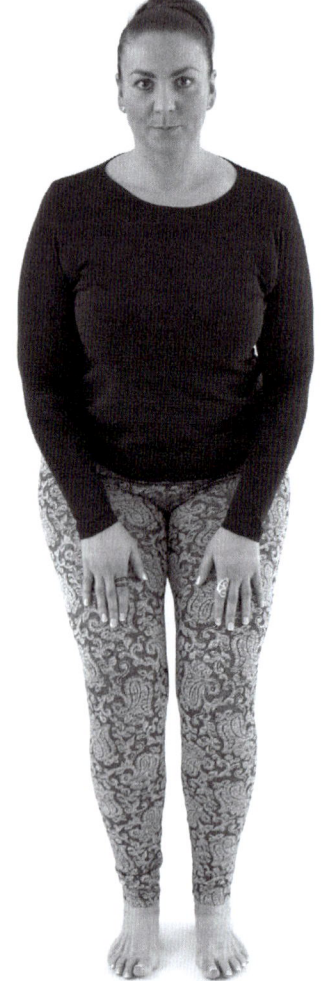
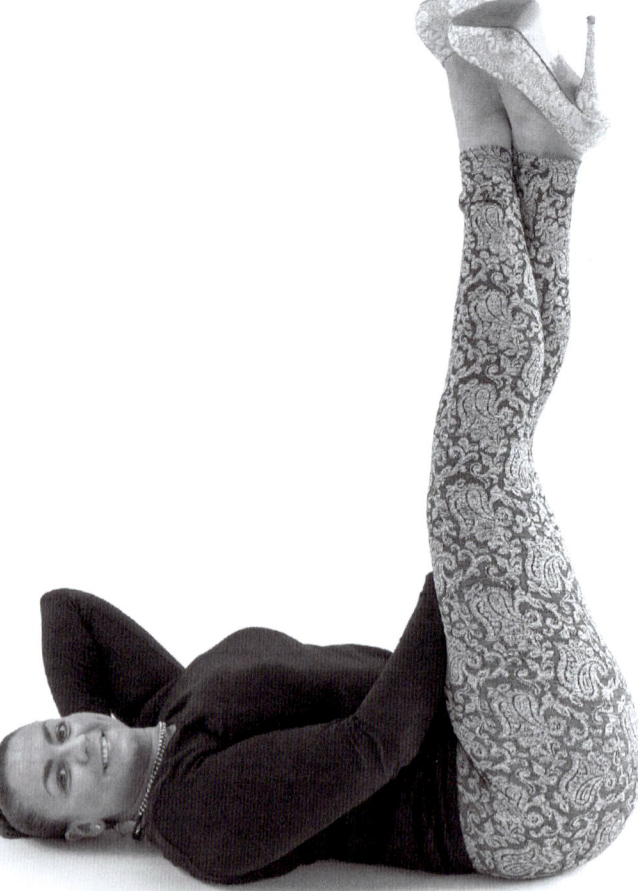

Standing Knee Raise with Optional Leg Extension

Improving your balance will enable you to be more adventurous with your sexual positions. Remember your posture throughout.

Always maintain posture key points when performing standing exercises.

Purpose: To increase strength of legs and improve balance.

Bedroom Pleasure: Maintain sexual positions and increase ability to perform the more advanced positions.

Repetitions: Repeat up to 8-12 times.

1. Stand with your weight evenly distributed and lengthen through the legs, spine and neck. Gently squeeze your booty, keep the belly button drawn in.

2. Knee Lifts - Placing your weight onto one foot, lift the knee to hip level, maintaining tall through the spine, control the movement hold for a second and gently place the foot back down. Repeat.

3. Optional – Keeping the knee level with the hip and balancing on the supporting leg, extend at the knee and lengthen the leg. Hold before bending the knee and then placing the foot back to the floor.

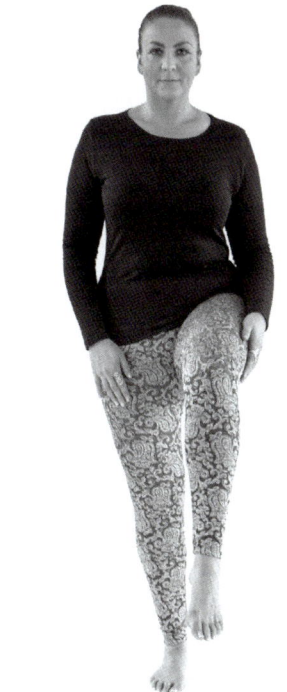

Show the world that you know you are beautiful where it counts.
Your self-confidence rises in direct proportion to your self-acceptance. Love the unique beautiful person that you are.

Checkpoints:

- You may need to have the knee lower than hip height to start.
- Ensure you breathe throughout.
- Watch the weight transfer, avoid pushing your weight to the opposite side.
- Think of using your booty as a brace, squeeze and firm your support base.

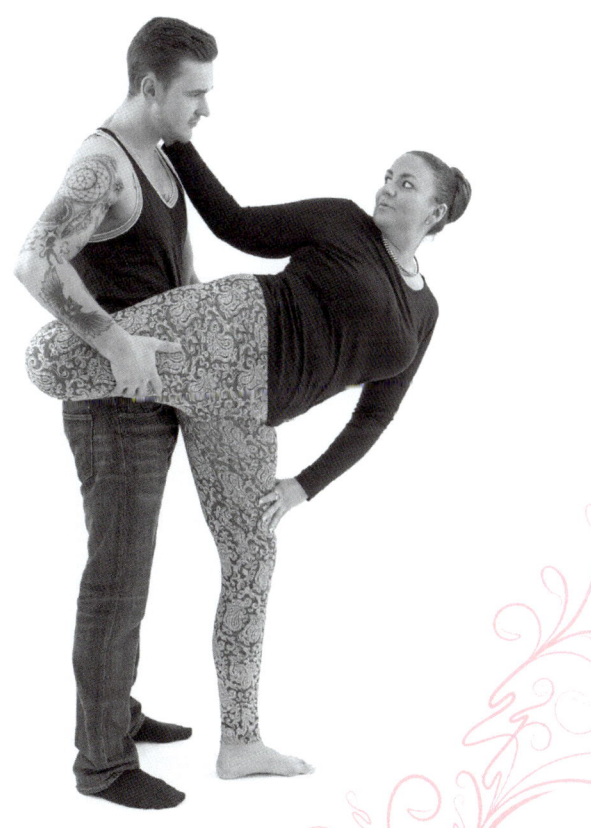

One Leg Balance

This exercise works both your balance and strength. With the hip open, the pelvic floor has to work that little harder. Improving your balance will enable you to be more adventurous with your sexual positions.

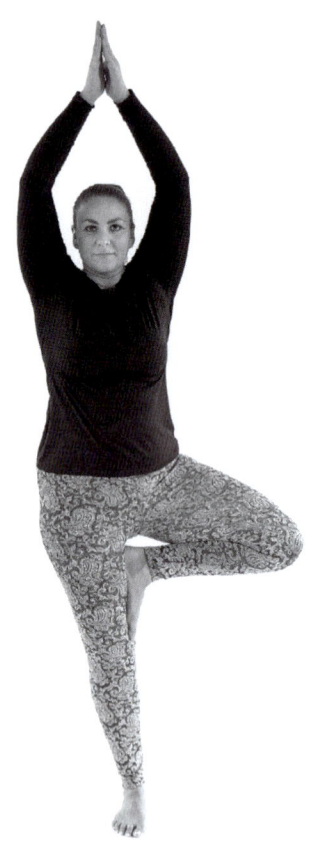

Purpose: To increase strength of legs and improve balance.

Bedroom Pleasure: Maintain sexual positions and increase ability to perform the more advanced positions.

Repetitions: Hold position for 10-30 seconds, 1-2 sets.

1. Stand with your weight evenly distributed and lengthen through the legs, spine and neck. Gently squeeze your booty, keep the belly button drawn in.

2. Rest the heel of one foot on the opposite leg, toes in contact with the floor, knee turned out to the side, making sure the movement comes from the hip.

3. To challenge the balance, rest the flat of the foot on the opposite lower leg, knee turned out to the side.

4. Hardest challenge is to rest the flat of the foot on the opposite inner thigh, knee turned out to the side. Tip: Press the foot firm into the inner thigh and the inner thigh into the foot.

5. Take the hands palms together above your head and hold.

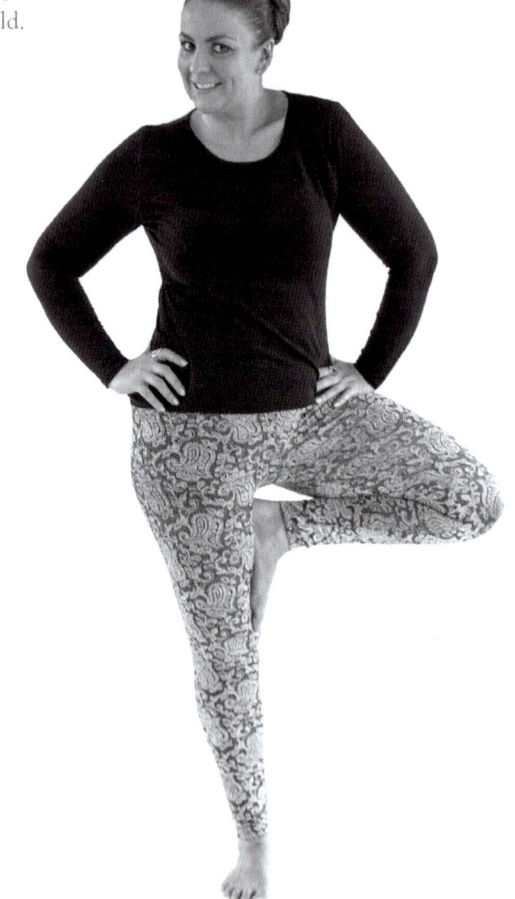

Checkpoints

- *Ensure you breathe throughout.*
- *Gradually build up the time you hold the position for.*

Bend Me Over with Optional Leg Lift

We take the deep stretch and add flowing movement to make this a great all over strength exercise.

Purpose: To strengthen the whole body and increase movement through the hips.

Bedroom Pleasure: This position can transfer straight to the bedroom.

Repetitions: Repeat up to 8-12 times.

1. Start in the all fours position, let your toes curl under, gently raise knees off the floor. Hold before taking a deep breathe in. As you exhale, push through your hands and lift your booty to the ceiling.

2. You are looking for a V shape ankle, knee and hip in alignment, hip, shoulder, elbow and wrist.

3. Once in position, press your heels towards the floor and drive your chest towards your thighs, keeping the booty on show.

4. Extend your right leg to the ceiling, take the option to open through the hip and hold for a few seconds before returning to the V shape, then down to knees hovering off the floor or back onto all fours before repeating on the other side.

Checkpoints

- *Remember the breathing, it is tempting to want to hold the breath.*
- *If you need to soften through the knees take the option.*
- *The leg lift is optional.*

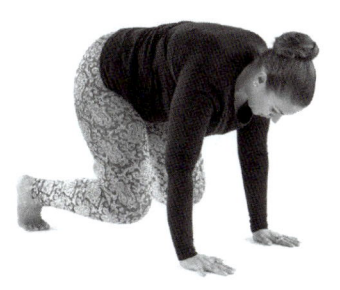
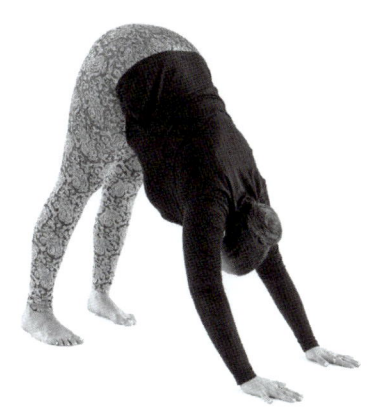
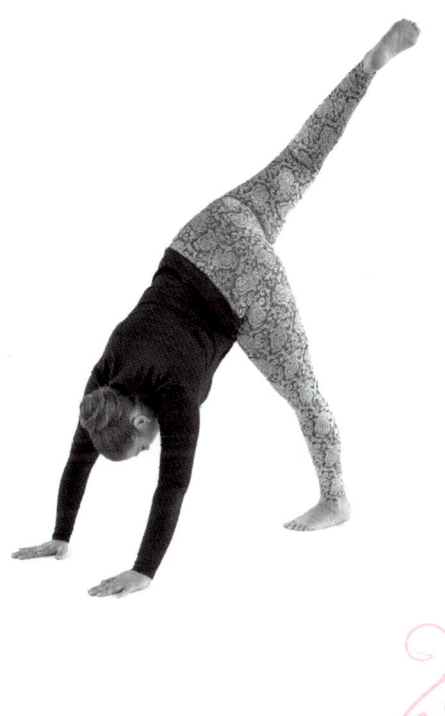
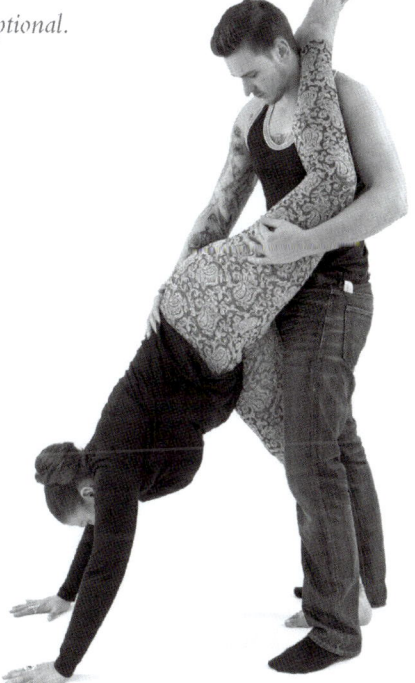

On All Fours

Working from an all fours position, the opposite arm and leg lift challenges the core and balance. Strengthening the body allowing full control. The adapted version of this exercise is one of the pure Pilates exercises it is a great starting point and over time you can progress and add variety.

Purpose: To increase core awareness and control.

Bedroom Pleasure: Improved awareness of your body allows for greater satisfaction.

Repetitions: Repeat up to 8-12 times.

1. Kneeling on all fours. Consider the key points for the All Fours position. You may prefer to rest on your knuckles opposed to your palms on the floor.

2. Keep the belly button pulled into the spine as you breathe out extend your right leg and your left arm. You are aiming to keep the hip, knee and ankle in alignment, shoulder elbow and wrist. Be aware not to rotate through the shoulders or the hips.

3. Repeat on the other side. If you need to perform the exercise with just the arms or just the legs extending please take this option. If your wrists feel under too much strain come down onto your forearms and work through the legs only.

4. An advanced option – The Opener; maintaining the knee level with your hip and your elbow with your shoulder reach behind to touch your foot before returning to the midline and then repeating on the other side.

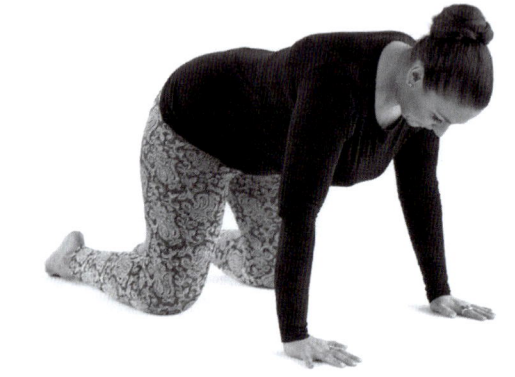

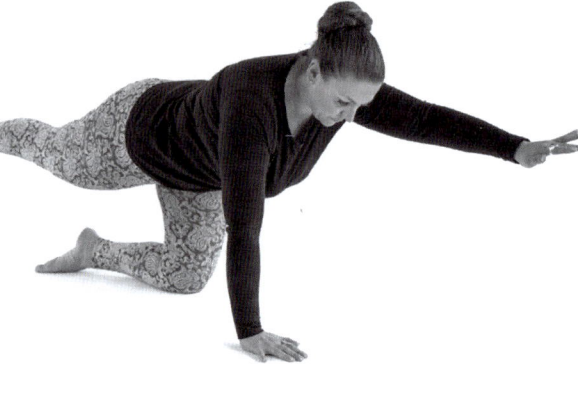

Checkpoints

- *Use the breathing to increase the range of movement. Think about breathing out (exhale) on the effort.*

- *Ease through the movement, always stay under control.*

- *Watch you do not drop through the lower back, draw the belly button in, hips tucked under, limit the rotation.*

- *To help keep the focus on stabilising through the back consider four glasses of wine resting on your back, one on each shoulder blade and one either side of the lower back. Do not spill the wine this you will need for the bedroom!*

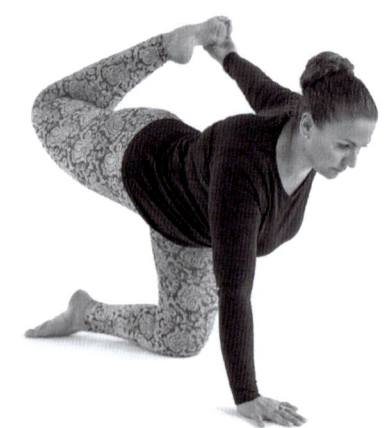

Extended Arm Plank (Push Up)

This is a classic exercise for shaping the upper body: the shoulders and arms. If it is performed properly your core will get a workout too.

In every position, pull the belly button in, always think of using your core, and keep your spine in neutral. Check for tension in your neck. There is no rush do what version is right for you and build up gradually to the full push-up.

Purpose: To strengthen the upper body.

Bedroom Pleasure: To be able to hold your body weight over your parter and seduce.

Repetitions: Repeat up to 8-12 times.

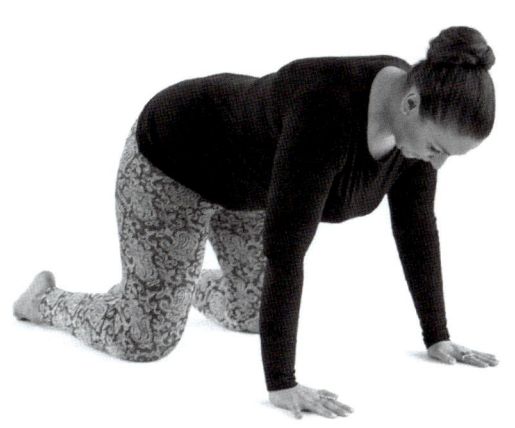 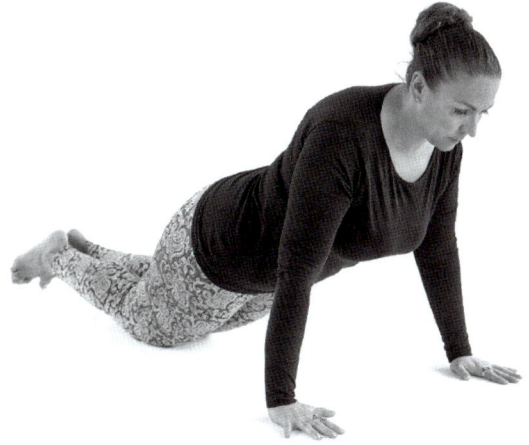

1. Position yourself on all fours, knees directly under your hips and hands directly under your shoulders, with the fingertips facing forwards. Keep your spine in neutral and keep your eyes to the floor, no tension through the neck.

2. Keeping your head in line with your spine, exhale as you lower your chest to the floor between your hands by bending your elbows. Be aware of your core. As you push up, straighten the arms without locking the elbows.

---

1. Drop your hips so that there is a straight line from your head to your knees. Your fingertips should be facing forwards and hands directly under the shoulders. Keep the core strong and your hips square.

2. Exhale as you lower. Keep your head in line with your spine and forward of your hands. Keep your weight evenly distributed between your knees and your hands.

Checkpoints

- *Do not lock the elbows.*
- *Lower only as far as you can control.*
- *Keep your chest at hand level and your head forward of your hands.*

Checkpoints

- *Keep a straight line from your head to your knees.*
- *Do not let your bottom stick up.*
- *Do not arch or curve your back.*

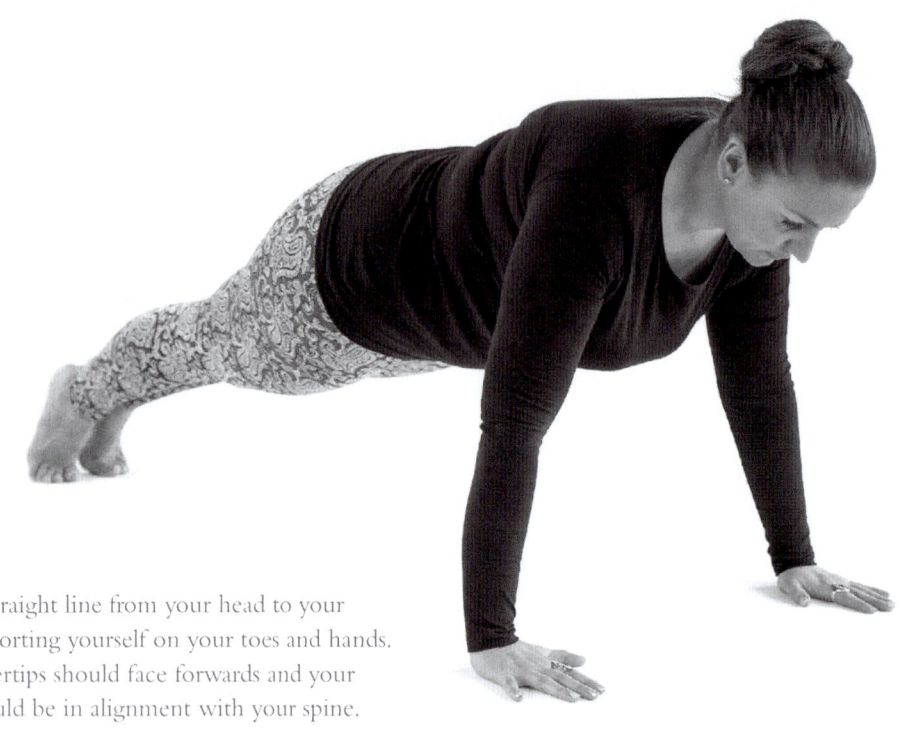

1. Form a straight line from your head to your feet, supporting yourself on your toes and hands. The fingertips should face forwards and your head should be in alignment with your spine.

2. Lower your chest to the floor between your hands, then push up, keeping your elbows soft. Keep the movement controlled and continuous. Lower only as far as you can control.

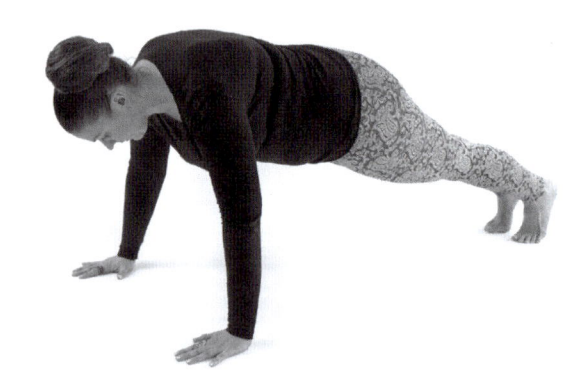

Checkpoints

- *Keep your shoulder blades down the spine.*
- *Make it a controlled, flowing movement.*
- *Breathe throughout.*

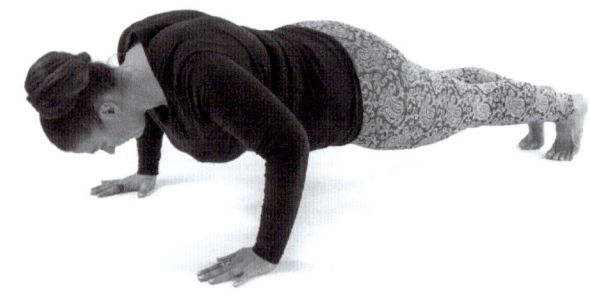

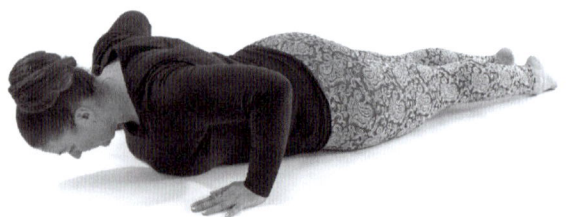

Full Body Hold (Plank)

A traditional exercise predominantly strengthening the core but also great for thighs and shoulders. Think about the pelvic floor tilt to really draw upon the deep core muscles.

Purpose: To strengthen the core.

Bedroom Pleasure: A strong core means you can hold many advanced sexual positions.

Repetitions: Hold for 10-30 seconds, 1-2 sets.

1. Drop your hips so that there is a straight line from your head to your knees. Gently place your forearms onto the mat, elbows under the shoulders. Keep the core strong.

2. As you hold this position ensure your weight is evenly distributed on your forearms and tilt the hips under, engage the pelvic floor.

3. The full hold on your toes will truly challenge the core, if you lower back feels agitated please stay on your knees. When on your toes you should be able to keep your booty level with your shoulders.

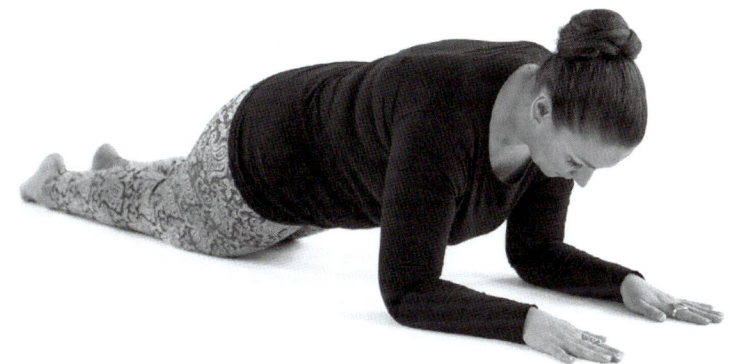

Checkpoints

- *Breathe throughout.*
- *Rest if you feel discomfort in your lower back.*

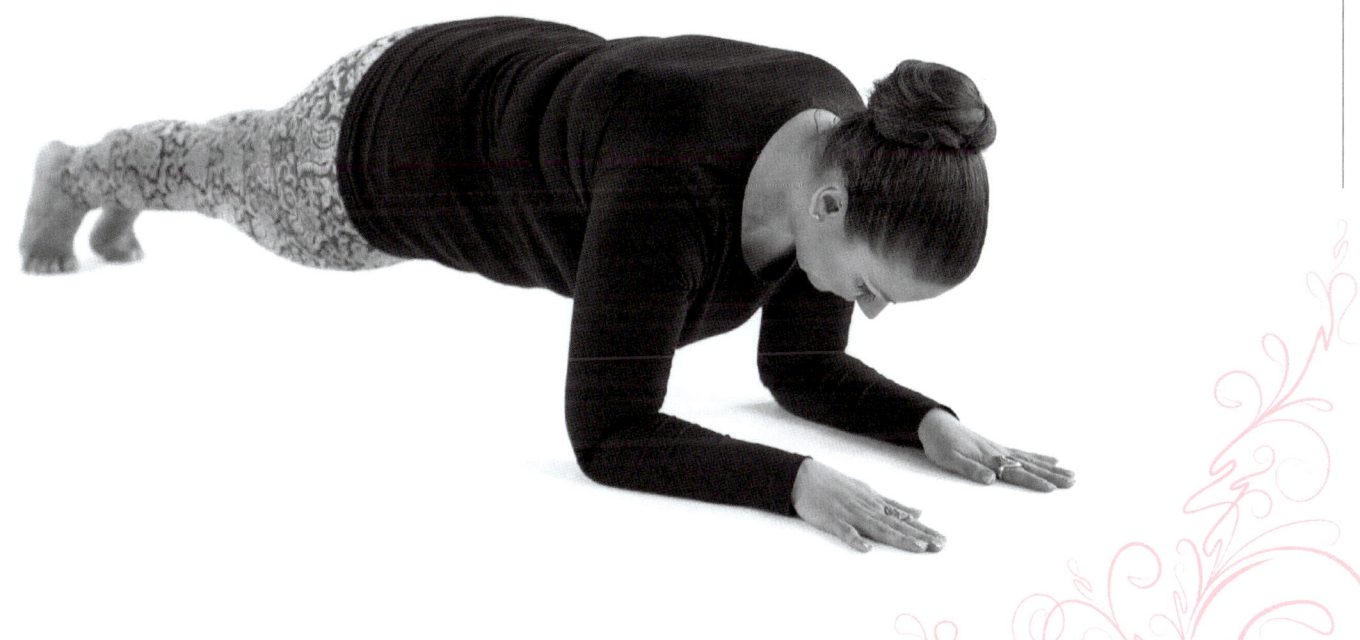

Lying on Front – Booty Brace

The Booty Brace allows you to really focus on the core and strengthening the lower body whilst under lengthened control. This move transfers straight to the bedroom, va va voom.

Purpose: To strengthen the booty.

Bedroom Pleasure: Increased movement and ability to hold this sexual position.

Repetitions: Hold 10–30 seconds, 1–2 sets.

1. Lying on your front, allow your hands to rest under your chin, or place your forehead on your heads to ensure neutral spine.

2. Keep the belly button pulled into the spine, legs long, gently squeeze your booty and hold. Ensure you breathe as opposed to holding your breath.

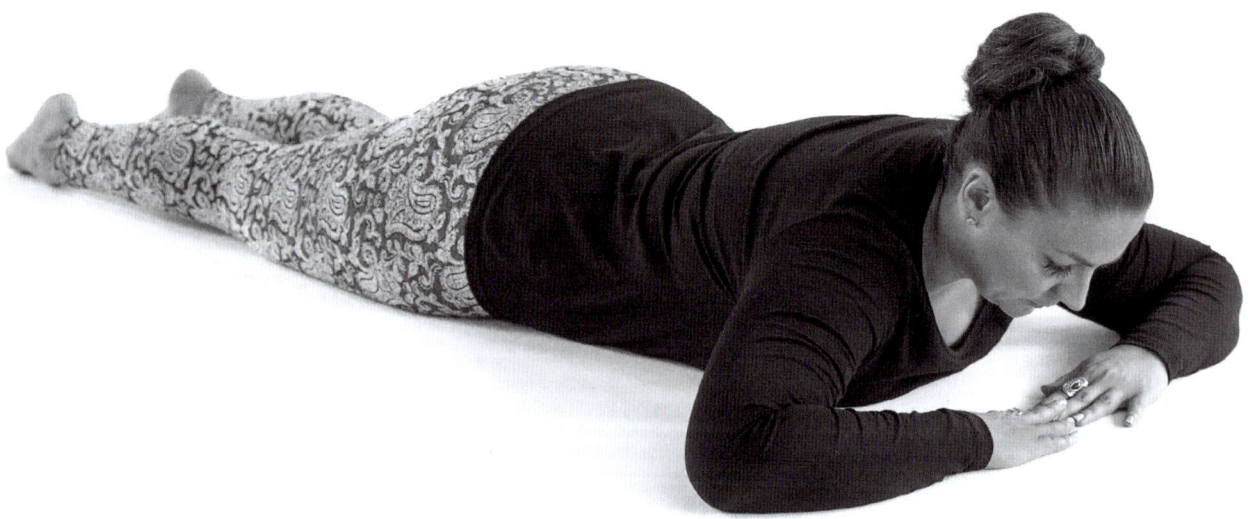

Checkpoints

- *Use the breathing to increase control and focus.*
- *Watch you do not drop through the lower back, draw the belly button in and hips tucked under.*

Opposite Arm & Leg

The opposite arm and leg lift whilst lying face down allows you to really focus on the core and strengthening of the whole body whilst under lengthened control.

Purpose: To increase core awareness and control.

Bedroom Pleasure: Improved awareness of your body allows for greater satisfaction.

Repetitions: Repeat up to 8-12 times.

1. Lying on your front in a booty brace, focus on pulling the belly button in and hips gently tucked under.

2. Keep the belly button pulled into the spine and as you breathe out, extend your right leg and your left arm. Be aware not to rotate through the shoulders or the hips.

3. Repeat on the other side.

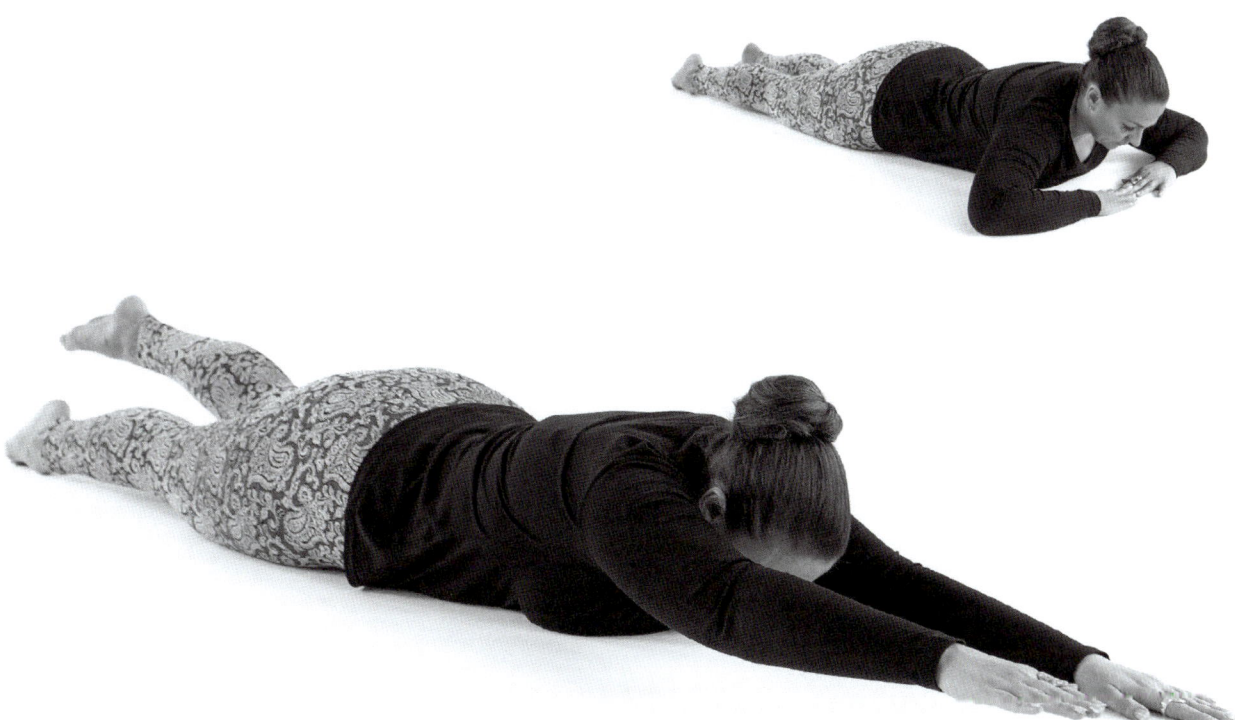

Checkpoints

- *Use the breathing to increase control and focus. Think about breathing out (exhale) on the effort.*
- *Watch you do not drop through the lower back, draw the belly button in, hips tucked up, limit the rotation.*

Squeeze & Lift

The Squeeze & Lift allows you to really focus on the core and strengthening of the lower body whilst under lengthened control. This exercise takes the Booty Brace to the next level.

Purpose: To strengthen the booty and legs.

Bedroom Pleasure: Increased stamina to hold positions.

Repetitions: Repeat up to 8-12 times.

1. Lying on your front, allow your hands to rest under your chin, or place your forehead on your hands to ensure neutral spine.

2. Keep the belly button pulled into the spine, legs long, gently squeeze your booty and hold. Ensure you breathe as opposed to holding your breath.

3. Lift one leg from the hip, keep the leg long and do not allow the core to relax, maintain awareness. Gently lower and repeat on the other side.

4. You can perform a double leg lift, ensure the lower back does not become over active. You can stretch at anytime.

5. With the leg lifts you can lift in the midline or out to the side to add variety.

6. I have also added a bent knee leg press, opposed to the leg lift, simply bend the knee and push the foot to the ceiling. Or why not try both feet together, knees open and press.

Checkpoints

- *Use the breathing to increase control and focus.*
- *Watch you do not drop through the lower back, draw the belly button in and hips tucked under.*
- *As your hips and spine increase in mobility and you gain strength through your booty and legs, you can take the move straight into the bedroom and enjoy.*

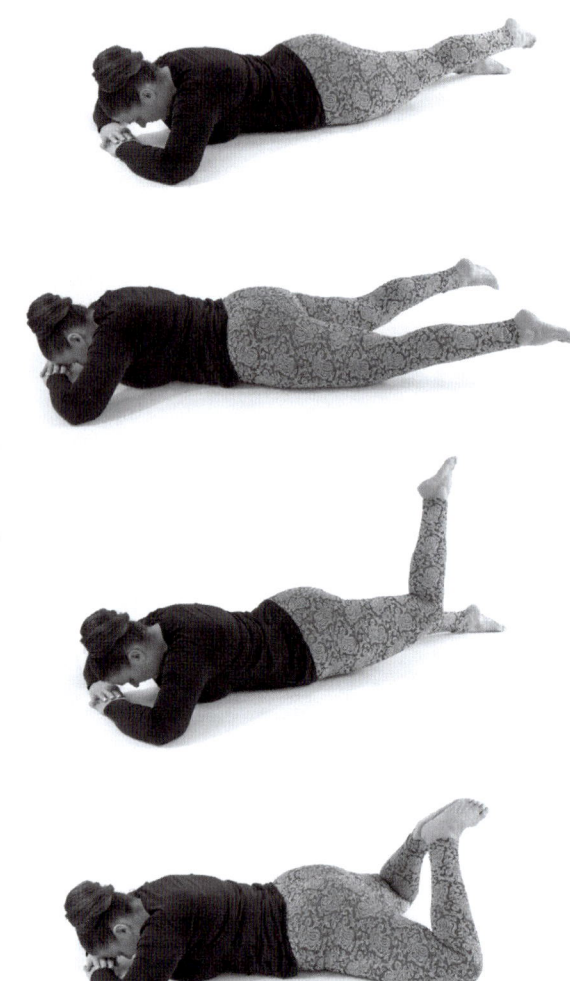

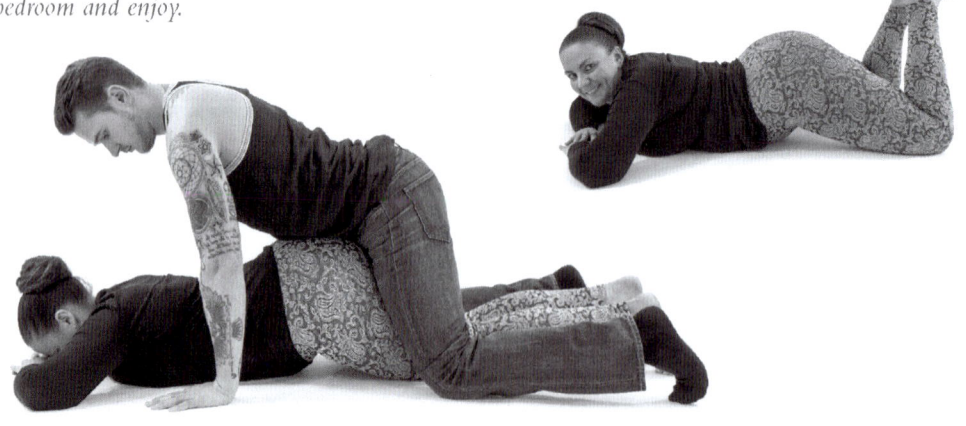

Arm Embrace

Earlier we took the Arm Embrace and performed standing. Here we take it lying down. Remember in the strength section we really focus on the draw down through the arms and visualise squeezing a grape through our shoulder blades to encourage the retraction, increase upper body strength and improve posture.

Purpose: To increase mobility and strength of upper body.

Bedroom Pleasure: Improved posture will mean you walk with more confidence.

Repetitions: Repeat up to 8-12 times.

1. Lying down in your Booty Brace, direct eyes to the floor to keep the spine neutral. Gently squeeze your backside and keep your belly button drawn in. Extend arms above your head and out to the side to form the shape of a V with your arms.

2. Drawing your elbows down to your waist, imagine you have a grape between your shoulder blades, retract the shoulder blades. Return to staring position and repeat.

3. Option to lift the upper body so you also work through the lower back.

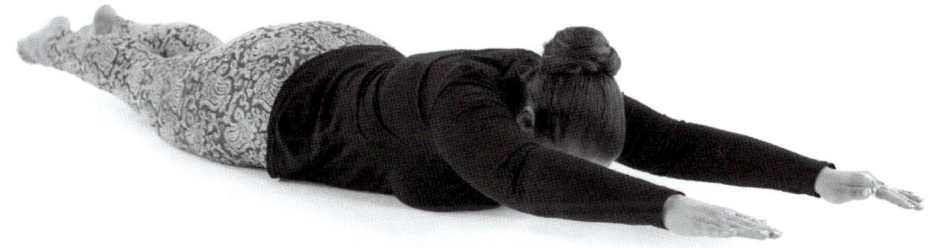

Checkpoints

- *Avoid tension through the neck.*
- *Breathe out as you pull the elbows into the waist.*

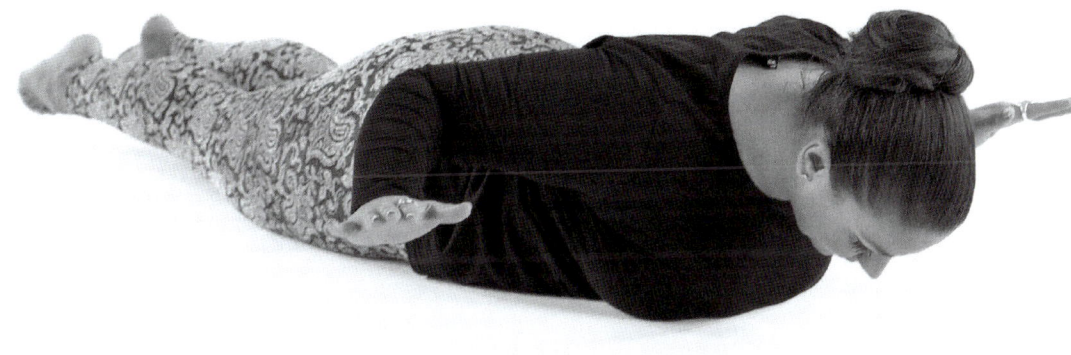

Side Lie – Side Hold (Side Plank)

A variation of the plank. Predominantly working the waistline.

Purpose: To strengthen the core/waistline.

Bedroom Pleasure: A strong core means you can hold many advanced sexual positions.

Repetitions: Hold for 10-30 seconds, 1-2 sets.

1. In a side lie position place one elbow under the shoulder and evenly distribute the weight on the forearm. Keep the core strong.

2. The bottom knee can stay fixed on the floor, bend the knee for greater stability. Imagine your partner has come and lifted your hips, pushing them up towards the ceiling. You can keep the top hand in front for support or extend the arm to the ceiling.

3. Staying in the side lie to increase the intensity, extend both legs. You can choose to stagger your feet or stack one foot on top of the other.

Checkpoints

- *Breathe throughout.*
- *Really press the hips towards the ceiling.*

Seated – Roll Back

I love the roll back, the base move for many advanced moves and gives the key to unlock full roll ups or often referred to as the traditional sit up.

Purpose: To mobilise the back and strengthen the abdominals.

Bedroom Pleasure: Increased stamina and unlock many positions.

Repetitions: Repeat up to 8-12 times.

1. Sit with your spine in neutral and your knees bent with both feet flat on the floor. Place your hands near your hips with your fingers facing your feet. Natural breathing, draw your belly button in towards your spine. Lower your chin towards your chest, then, using your hands for support, start to roll down to the floor.

    Try to place each vertebra on the floor, one by one. To do this, tilt your pelvis and curve your spine into a C-shape.

2. Once you have rolled down as far as you find comfortable, exhale and using your core strength, return to the starting position. Pull up through the top of your head to create a long spine, then repeat. Use your arms only as support and avoid transferring all your weight onto the back of your arms.

Checkpoints

- *Keep your feet flat on the floor.*
- *Lengthen up through the spine at the end of the movement.*
- *Take care not to tense or grip around your neck.*

Rocker with Optional Raunch

Think about the roll back, we take it half way, control through the core, slowly lift our feet and hold. We can add so much variety and mastering the balance allows for adventure in the bedroom.

Purpose: Challenge the core and balance.

Bedroom Pleasure: Increase blood flow to the pelvic floor, increasing sensitivity and improving sexual pleasure.

Repetitions: Repeat up to 8-12 times.

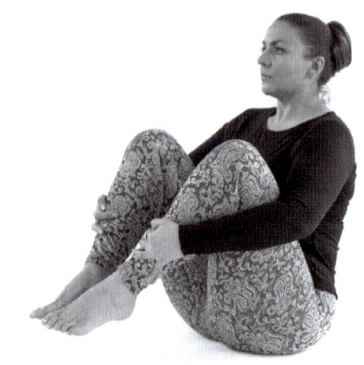

1. Sit with your spine in neutral and your knees bent with both feet flat on the floor. Place your hands near your hips with your fingers facing your feet. Inhaling wide and full through the ribs, draw your navel towards your spine. Lower your chin towards your chest, then, using your hands for support, gently lean back, keeping your shoulders retracted and spine long.

2. Lift your feet off the floor and hold gently, knees bent. Avoid the temptation to round the shoulders.

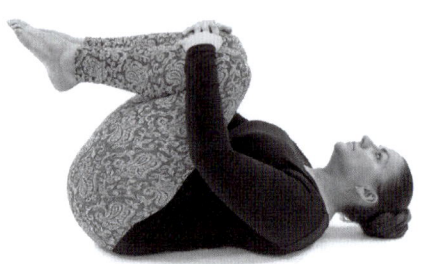

3. Under control as you breathe out, roll back to the floor and at the bottom, take a deep breath in. As you exhale, roll back up to the starting position. Optional to hover your feet as you come back up.

4. From the photo you will see what I have termed the 'raunch'. As you come back up seated under control lengthen one or both legs. You can lengthen to the front or to the sides, now we all know where this will lead. Gain the confidence to hold this position and feel how the bedroom activities heat up.

Checkpoints

- *Lengthen up through the spine, lift your chest.*
- *Take care not to tense around your neck and shoulders.*

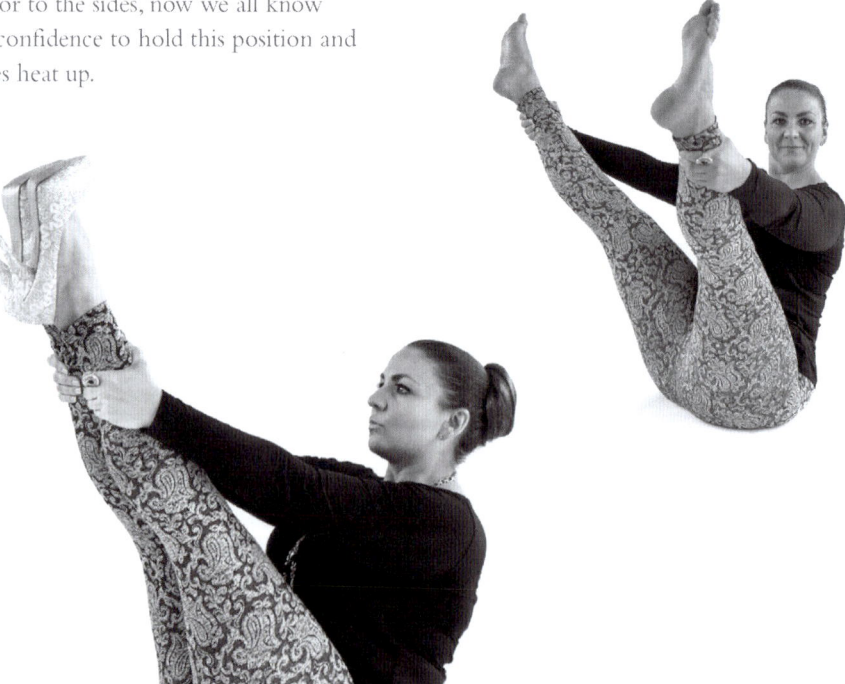

On Your Back - Table Top Tease

An excellent core stabiliser and strengthener, your tummy muscles will really feel this! As you hold for as long as comfortable, it is a great way to strengthen the core without movement. The movement can cause discomfort especially if you have a lower back condition so a great exercise to perfect.

Purpose: To strengthen the core.

Bedroom Pleasure: Strong core means ability to experiment in the bedroom and also take control of your orgasm.

Repetitions: Hold for 10-30 seconds, 1-2 sets.

1. Lie on your back with your arms by your sides, slide your shoulder blades down your spine and lengthen your arms away. Bring your knees level with your hips and feet in line with knees (imagine you are resting your feet on a chair), your head and spine in neutral.

   If you find lifting both knees causes discomfort, please alternate the legs and hold each for a couple of seconds before switching.

2. As you hold the position draw the belly button down towards the mat. Ensure you control the breathing and make sure the knees stay in line with the hips.

3. To make it harder you could take the feet and inch or two away from the body and lift the head and shoulders avoiding dropping the chin to the chest.

Checkpoints

- *Control your breathing.*
- *If you feel your back arching, rest, relax, stretch and repeat.*
- *Remember the option to alternate the legs.*

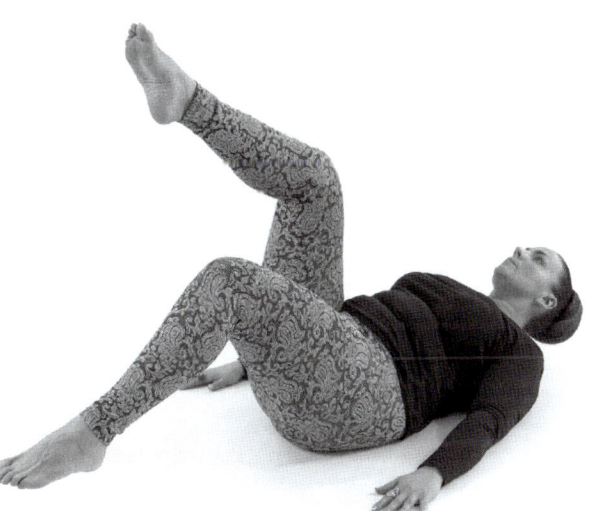

Please visit **www.pilatesforbettersex.com** for more ideas on routines for all levels.

Sexy Scissor Switch

Strengthen the lower tummy muscles and feel the lengthening through your legs. You can really get into a rhythm and synchronise your breathing with each movement. Imagine the sexual positions you are able to get into with mobile hips, lengthened thighs and a controlled core.

Purpose: To strengthen core and stretch the back of the thighs.

Bedroom Pleasure: Use your legs to get into various positions and also wrap round your partner and hold firm.

Repetitions: Repeat 8–12 times.

1. Lie on your back with your arms by your sides, slide your shoulder blades down your spine and lengthen your arms away. Tilt your pelvis and lengthen the tailbone away. The whole length of your spine should be in contact with the floor.

2. Bring one knee into the chest and gently hold over the top of the knee or under the thigh. Keep the belly button in towards the mat lift the opposite leg a couple of inches off the floor.

3. As you exhale, switch legs drawing the other knee into the chest. Keep the movement flowing – optional to lift the head and shoulders off the mat but avoid tension through the neck.

4. An advanced position, extend the leg of the bent knee to the ceiling. Both legs long, complete the full leg switch and uniform the breathing.

Checkpoints

- *Ensure the movement flows.*
- *Breathe throughout.*

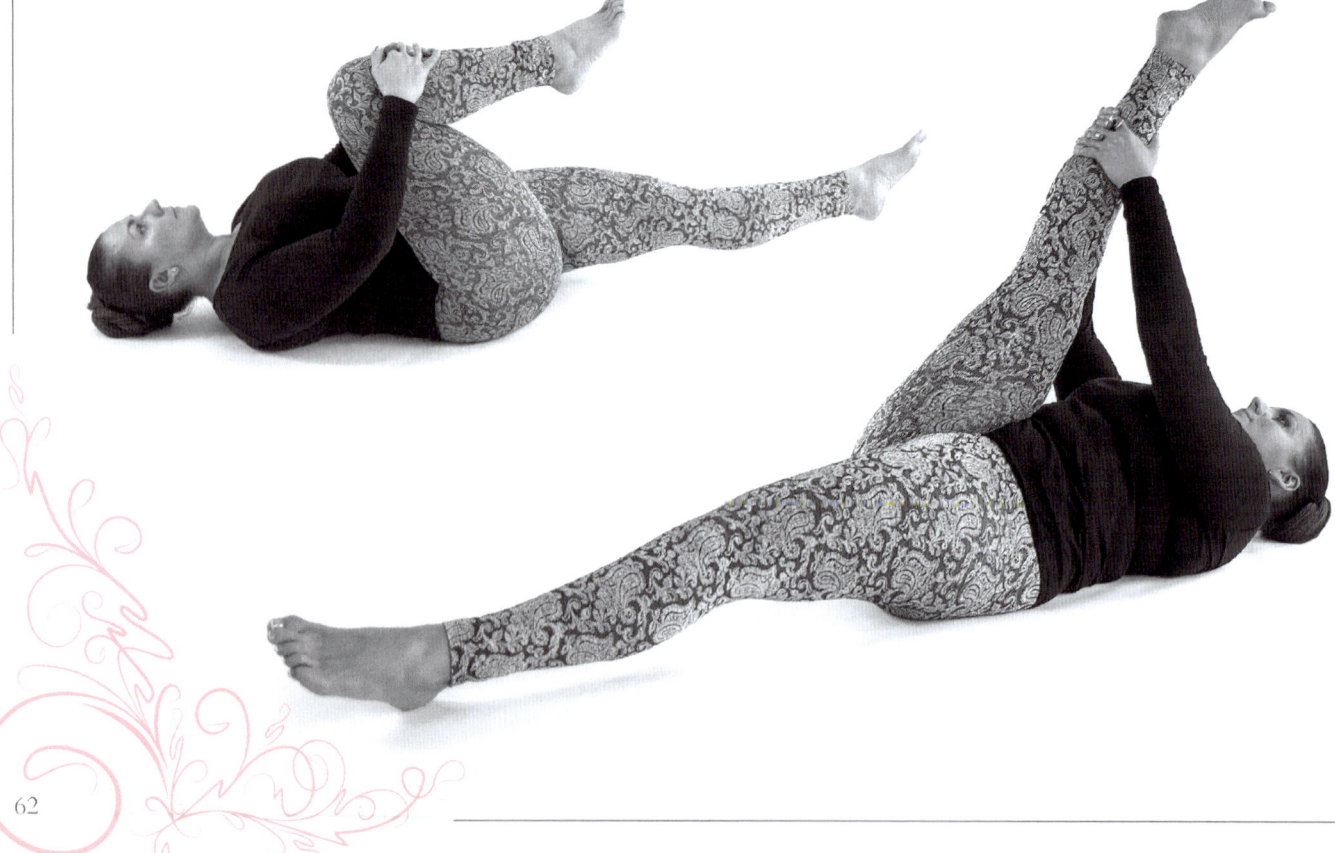

Shoulder Booty Bridge

This is a great mobiliser which will loosen a stiff back & increase blood flow to the pelvic area. The aim is for each bone in your spine to lift off the floor in succession. You may find that, to begin with, your back lifts in two or three sections: try to create length between each vertebra. As you lower yourself, place each vertebra in turn on the floor.

The hips should be perfectly level and you should try to create as much distance between your hips and your shoulders as possible. Do not forget to tilt the pelvis as you begin the movement. To mobilise the spine fully, be sure to return to neutral as you lower your back to the floor, just before you tilt the pelvis and start the next lift.

Purpose: To mobilise the spine, challenge the abdominals and strengthen the booty.

Bedroom Pleasure: Increase blood flow to the pelvic floor, increasing sensitivity, improving sexual pleasure.

Repetitions: Repeat 8-12 times.

1. Lie on your back with your arms by your sides, slide your shoulder blades down your spine and lengthen your arms away. Bend your knees and place your feet hip width apart, flat on the mat. Your head is in alignment and your spine, in neutral.

2. Tilt your pelvis and lengthen the tailbone away. The whole length of your spine should be in contact with the floor.

3. Slowly peel your spine up off the floor bone by bone, raising your hips towards the ceiling and keeping the abdominals flat and drawn down. Make the movement smooth and flowing. Once you get used to the movement you can increase the stretch by taking your arms over your head.

Checkpoints

- *Keep the hips level.*
- *Maintain the distance between the hips and the ribs.*
- *Make the movement flow.*

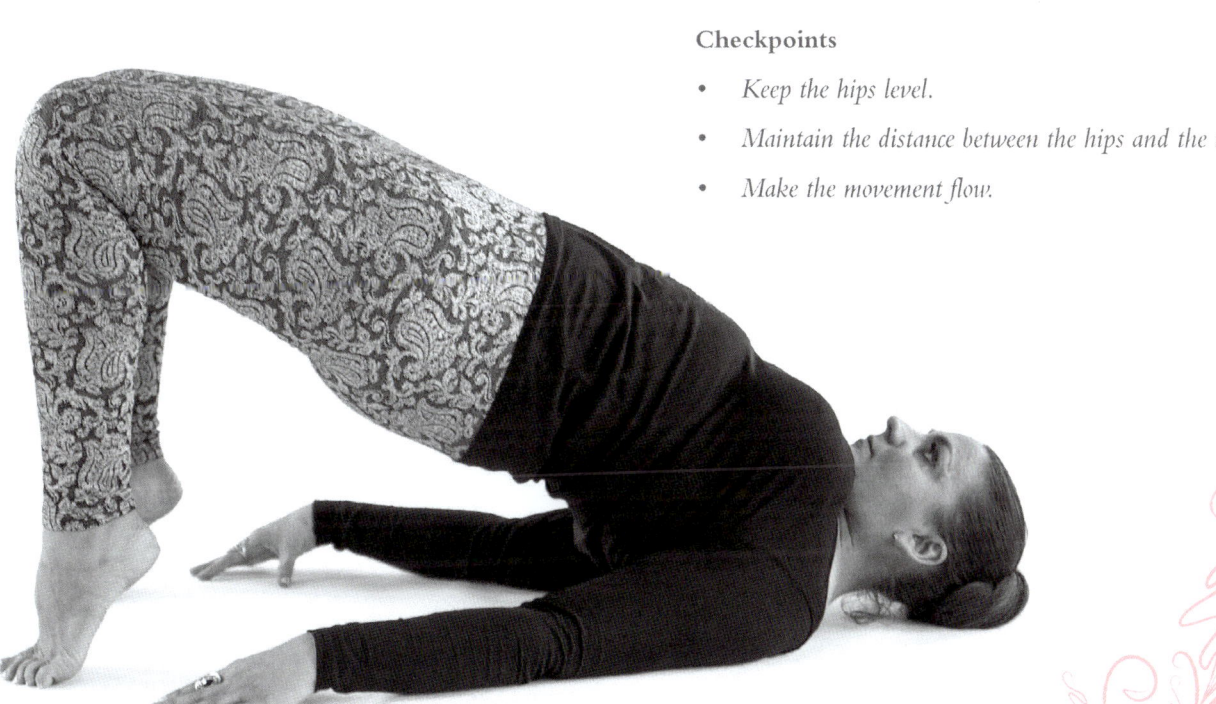

Flirt with the Flip

This is an advanced move and to hold this position during sexual pleasure, is a skill but also very fun. You can experiment and wrap your legs around your partner or even have your partner support your weight.

Purpose: To strengthen the whole body.

Bedroom Pleasure: Increased stamina to hold positions, get real freaky.......

Repetitions: Repeat 8-12 times.

1. Lying on your front, place your palms by the sides of your chest.

2. Keep the belly button pulled into the spine, legs long. Bend the right knee and push foot to the ceiling, take the leg over to the opposite side and come up seated.

3. When you are seated your right foot should be flat to the floor and your left leg straight, your left hand pressed to the floor arm extended.

4. Driving through the left hand and right foot lift your booty, pressing the hips to the ceiling. Hold then slowly release and practice on the other side.

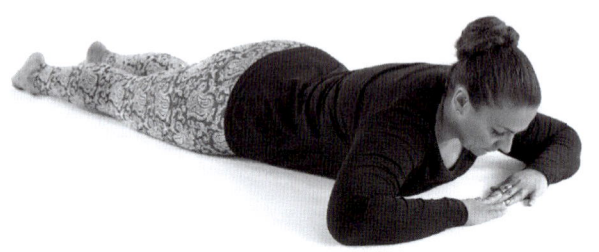
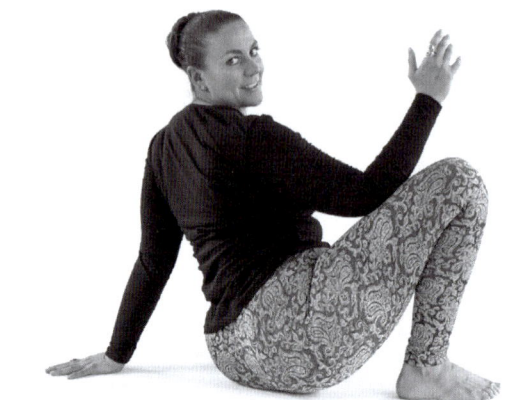
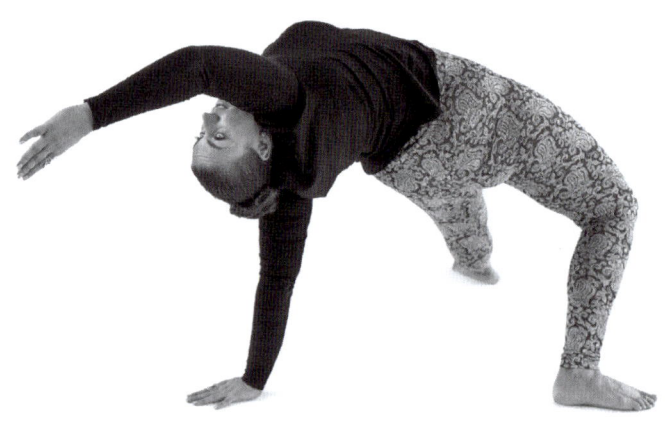
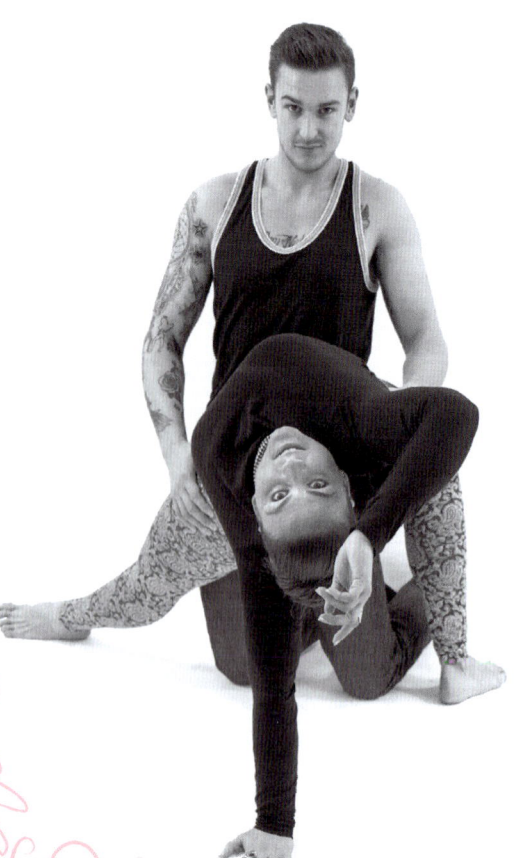

Checkpoints

- Use the breathing to increase control and focus.
- Part 4 is optional, you can stay with parts 1-3 and build up to part 4.

Let It Flow – Beginner

Visit **www.pilatesforbettersex.com** for more ideas on routines for all levels.

Arm Embrace	44
Tight Legged Squat	46
Booty Brace	54
Opposite Arm & Leg	55
Arm Embrace	44
Roll Back	59
Booty Bridge	63

Let It Flow - Intermediate

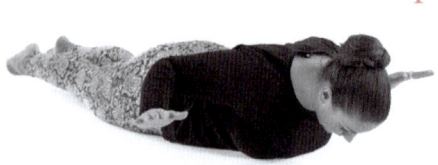

Visit **www.pilatesforbettersex.com** for more ideas on routines for all levels.

Arm Embrace	57
Squeeze & Lift	56
Push Up	51
Full Body Hold	53
Bend Me Over	49
Wide Leg Press	45

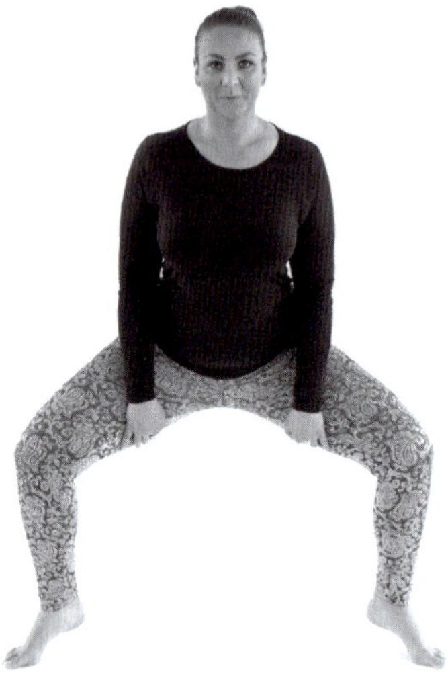

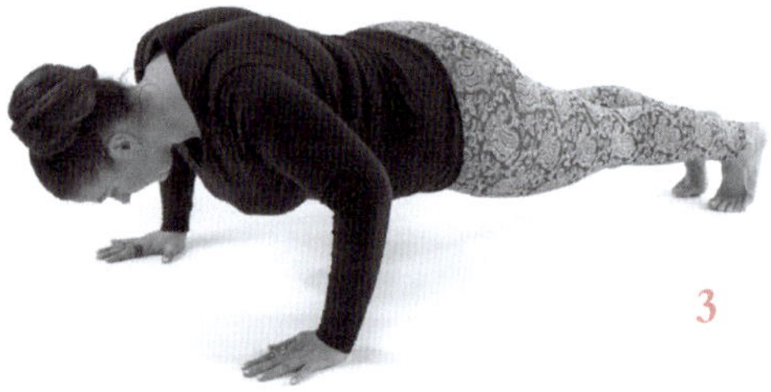

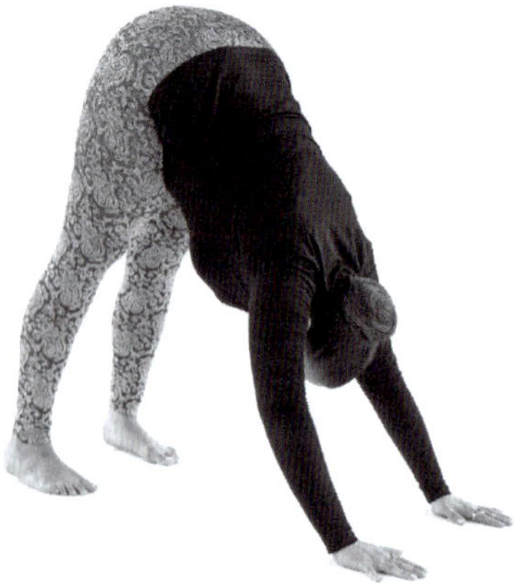

1

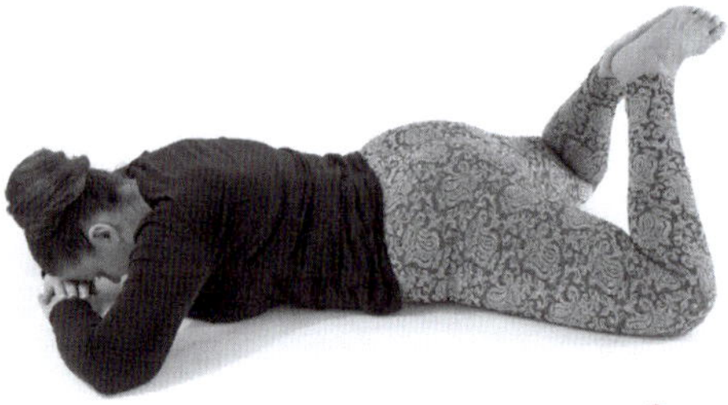

2

6

3

5

4

Visit **www.pilatesforbettersex.com** for a more advanced routine

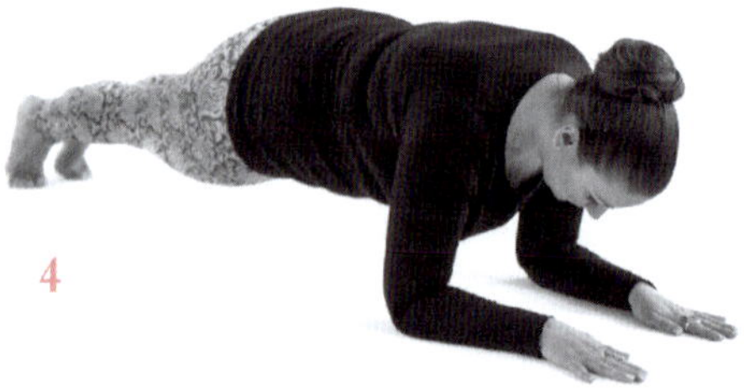

Chapter 5

Increase Flexibility for Deeper Enjoyment

Standing – Roll Down

This practices flowing movement and challenges the stomach muscles to control the spine. Teaches you to breathe with movement, relax into positions and respond to your body. As you perform the roll down, you will become aware of where you hold tension and where your body may resist certain movements or positions. Learn to let go and flow.

Purpose: Learn to flow and respond to your body. Release tension in the back of thighs.

Bedroom Pleasure: When you can respond to your body you transfer the skills to the bedroom.

Repetitions: Repeat up to 8-12 times or reduce the repetitions and enjoy the stretch at the bottom.

1. Stand with your feet slightly apart in your natural stance. Your spine should be neutral, neither arched nor tucked under. Feel the movement coming from your core.

2. As you breathe out, scoop the belly, nod the nose down, and peel the spine down to the floor: first the head, then the shoulders. Arms hang loose, let the arms drop fall towards the floor.

3. Roll the spine as far as you can without allowing the tail bone to rise up. Keep the pelvis upright. Breathe in. Then breathe out and gently peel back to standing position.

4. As an option, you can roll down half way and support your weight on your thighs and gently alternate a knee bend. Press the knee gently forward, lifting the heel and repeat on the other side.

Checkpoints

- *If you feel strain in your neck or shoulders, build the movement up slowly until you have released all tension. Learn to let go of your arms and neck completely.*

- *Soften through the knees if your back of thighs are particularly tight. Flexibility will improve by following the programme.*

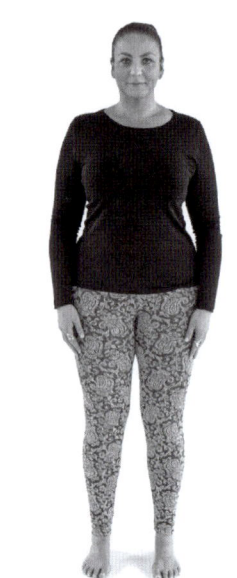
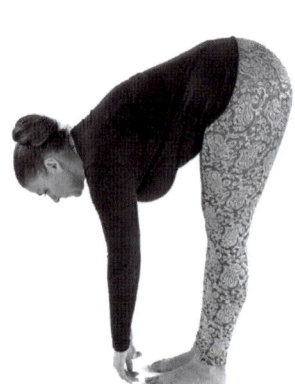
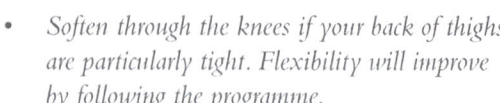

All Fours – Booty Release

This is a great stretch for reaching deep into your booty. I promise; get this right and it feels so good.

Purpose: To stretch and release the booty.

Bedroom Pleasure: Will mean more stamina and a booty you can control, which will drive him wild.

Repetitions: Hold for 10-30 seconds, 1-2 sets.

1. Kneeling on all fours. Position your hands under your shoulders and your knees under your hips. Spread your weight evenly. Pull the belly button in, gently tuck hips under.

2. Slide your right knee forward and your lower leg lies across the mat, gently ease your weight down, be careful of the knee joint.

3. You maybe able to slide the left leg further back, now support your weight through your upper body or simply relax into the stretch, lean forward and let it all go, take the stretch.

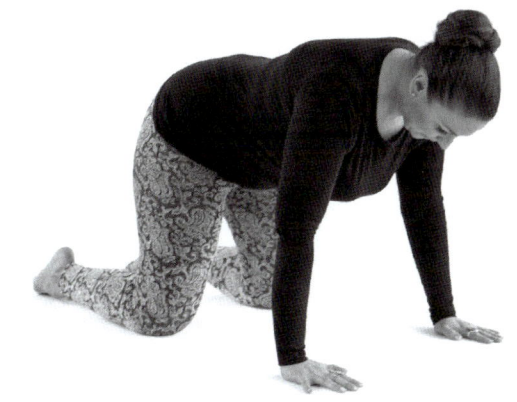

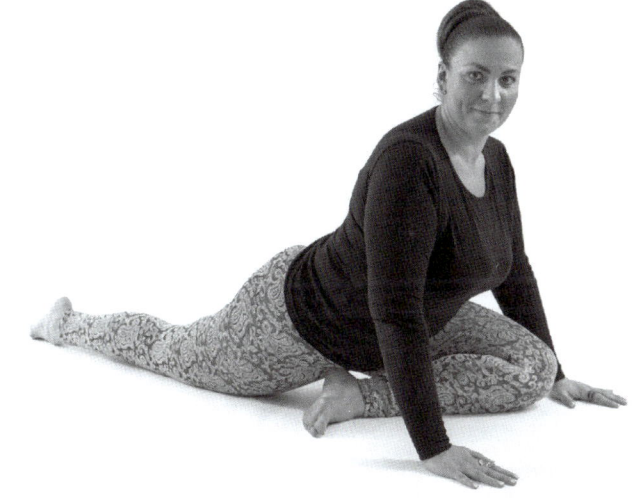

Checkpoints

- *Always breathe when holding stretches.*
- *Avoid the temptation to roll out of the stretch, keep weight central.*

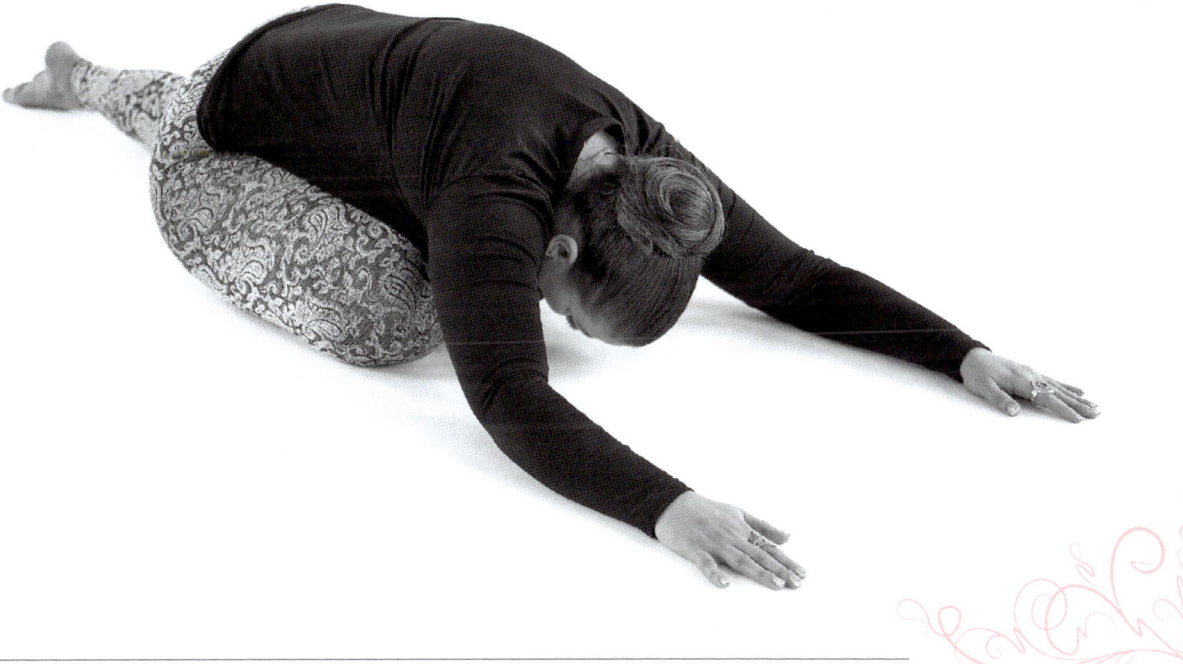

Shoulder Release

This is a great stretch for releasing the shoulders, increasing mobility through the trunk and stretching through the lower back. Below I have outlined a few variations.

Purpose: To stretch and release the upper body.

Bedroom Pleasure: Learn to breathe with the movement.

Repetitions: Hold for 10-30 seconds, 1-2 sets.

1. Kneeling on all fours. Position your hands under your shoulders and your knees under your hips. Spread your weight evenly. Pull the belly button in and gently tuck the hips under.

2. Take your right arm and thread underneath kissing the shoulder and your head to the floor. Really snuggle the waist round and hold.

3. As an option, the opposite arm and shoulder can open, come behind your back and rest the hand on the lower back or slide in contact with the inner thigh on the left leg. Really retract the shoulder back and ensure you do not hold your breath.

4. An option for those that like to flow the movements, repeat part 1-2; the right shoulder kissing the floor. Slide the left leg back and lift to the ceiling, keeping the limb long.

5. Pull the right arm back out and extend the arm to the ceiling at the same time lower the leg hover off the floor where possible. This really challenges the balance. Aim to perform a few repetitions on both sides.

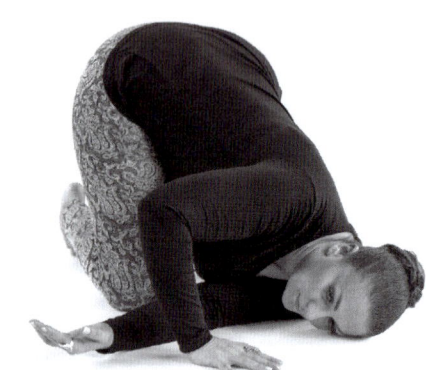

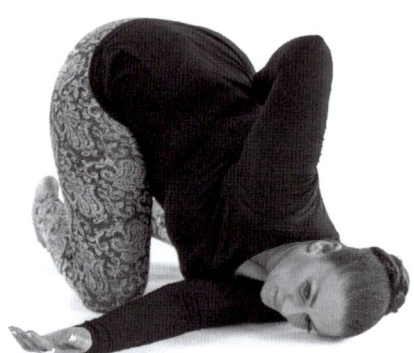

Checkpoints

- *Always breathe when holding stretches.*
- *The thread through with leg lift is advanced, please progress slowly.*

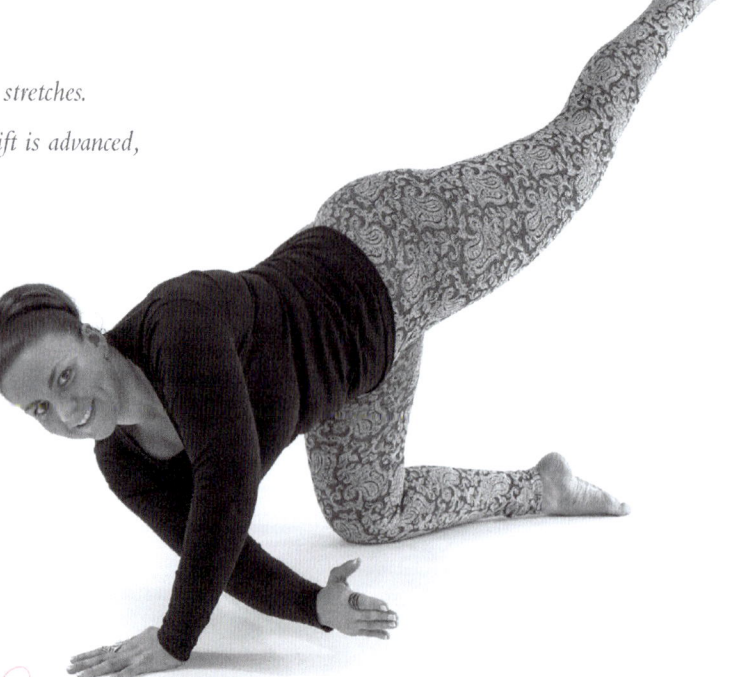

Curl & Release

Holding your body weight, being able to move your hips with ease and feel confident comes from the base exercise of the curl and release. This is a great starting point and over time you can progress to the strengthening exercises and/or stretches for deeper enjoyment.

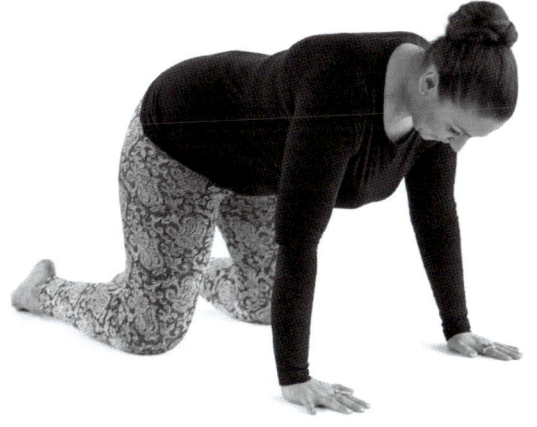

Purpose: To increase movement through the spine and hips.

Bedroom Pleasure: Builds strength enabling more advanced sexual positions.

Repetitions: Repeat up to 8-12 times.

1. Kneeling on all fours. Consider the key points for the All Fours position. Bring your chin to your chest and tuck the hips under, curling up through the spine. You may prefer to rest on your knuckles opposed to your palms flat to the floor.

2. Under control, tilt your tailbone to the ceiling, emphasising the booty whilst lifting the chest and looking forward.

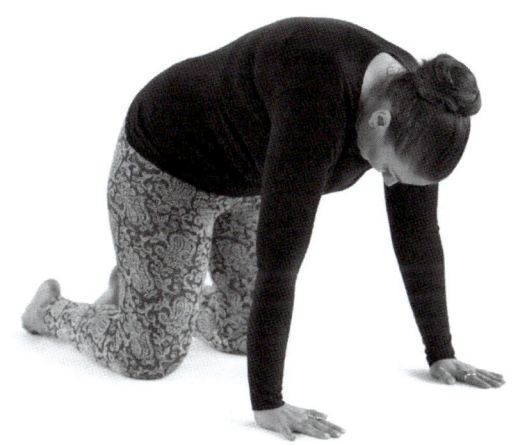

Checkpoints

- *Use the breathing to increase the range of movement. Think about breathing out (exhale) on the effort.*
- *Ease through the movement, stay under control.*

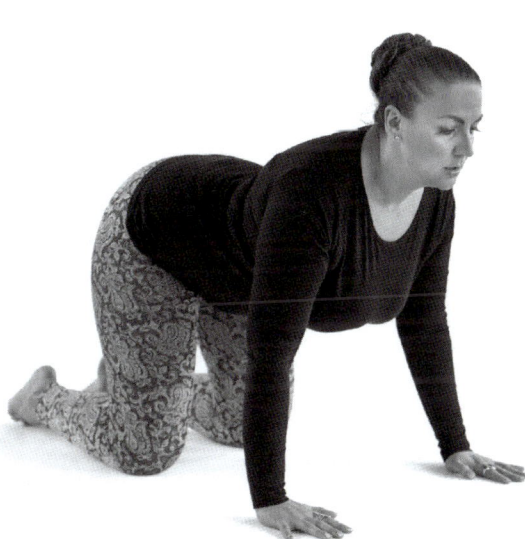

Be amazed at the wonder of your body. No matter your size, shape, or age, your body is a miraculous temple. It is home to you, a beautiful person, embrace your 'you'ness.

Sit Back & Hold

A great stretch for your lower back but also your shoulders, releasing tension and tightness.

Purpose: To stretch and release your back and shoulders.

Bedroom Pleasure: This position can transfer straight to the bedroom, lift your booty slightly, let your partner slide in. Bring your arms back to support your weight and away you go.

Repetitions: Hold for up to 20-30 seconds, repeat 1-2 times.

1. Start in the all fours position. Push your weight back towards your heels, with your arms reaching out in front.

2. If you prefer sit with your knees wide, push you weight back and aim to bring your chest towards the floor.

3. Another option is to reach for your heels and pull into a small ball.

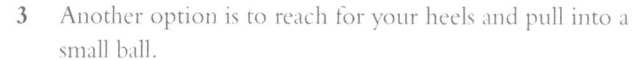

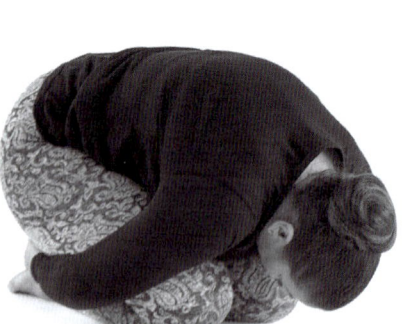

Checkpoints

- *Remember the breathing, it is tempting to want to hold the breath.*

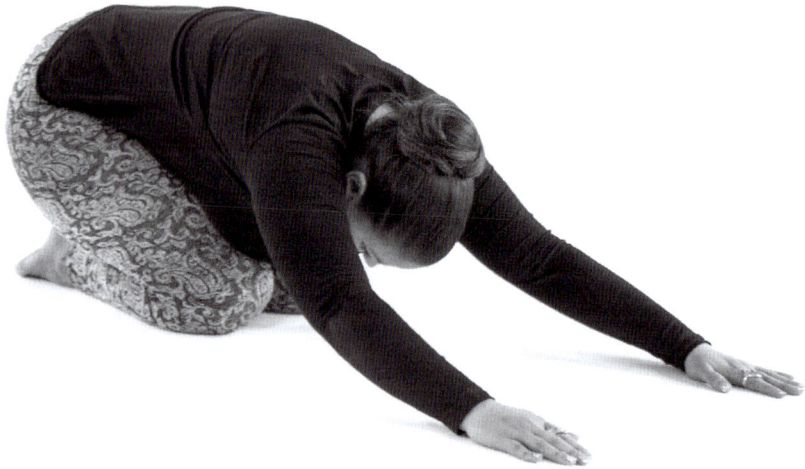

Seated – Inner Thigh Release

A great stretch for your inner thighs, I will go through two seated variations but note if you prefer the support for your lower back you can choose the lying down version as well.

Purpose: To stretch and increase flexibility of your inner thighs.

Bedroom Pleasure: Long and strong inner thighs means you can grip your partner tight.

Repetitions: Hold for up to 20-30 seconds, repeat 1-2 times.

1. Seating tall, lengthen through the spine, shoulders relaxed and back. Soles of your feet together.

2. Slowly allow the knees to drop towards the floor increasing the stretch of the inner thighs, breathe throughout.

3. Alternative open your legs wide, from the hips lean forward hands to the floor and hold the position. To increase the stretch take a deep breath in and as your exhale place your forearms to the floor.

4. If you prefer to lie on your back, bring your knees into your chest and hug into a small ball. Take the knees out to the side and reach for the ankles of heels and hold. Avoid tension through the neck.

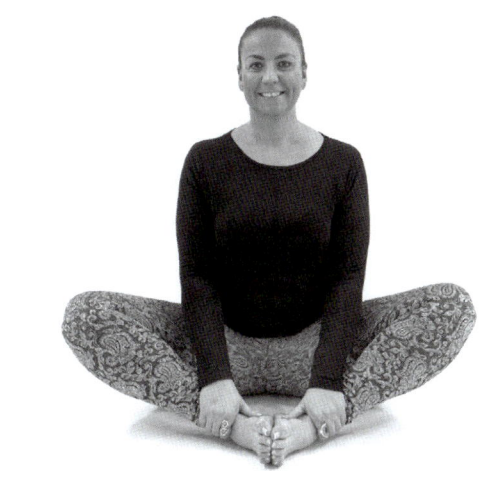

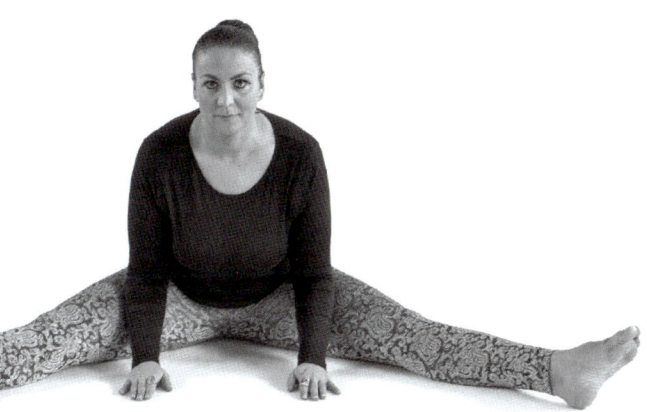

Checkpoints

- *Remember the breathing, it is tempting to want to hold the breath.*

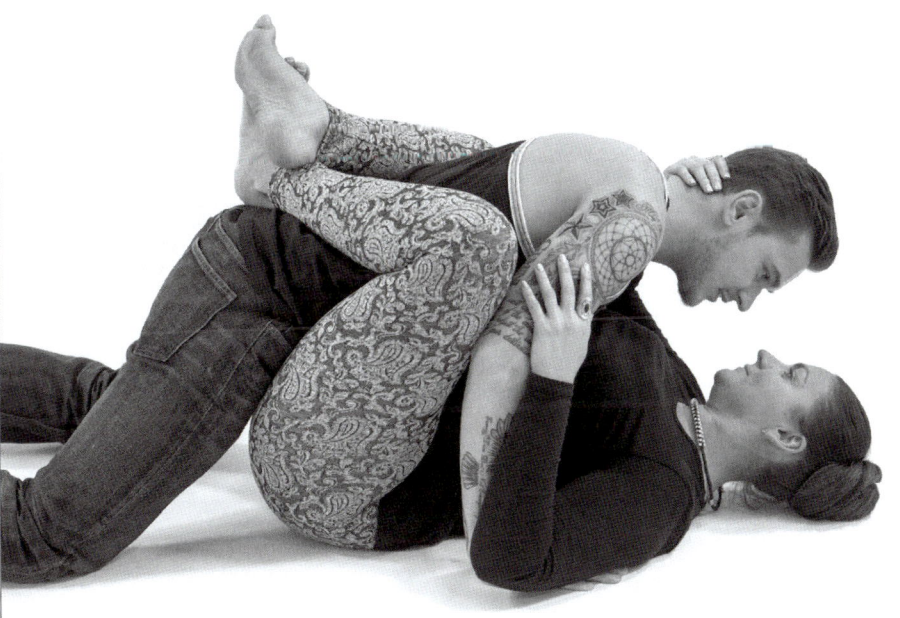

Lying on Front. - Front of Thigh Release

The Front of Thigh Release allows you to really focus on the core and lengthening the lower body whilst under control.

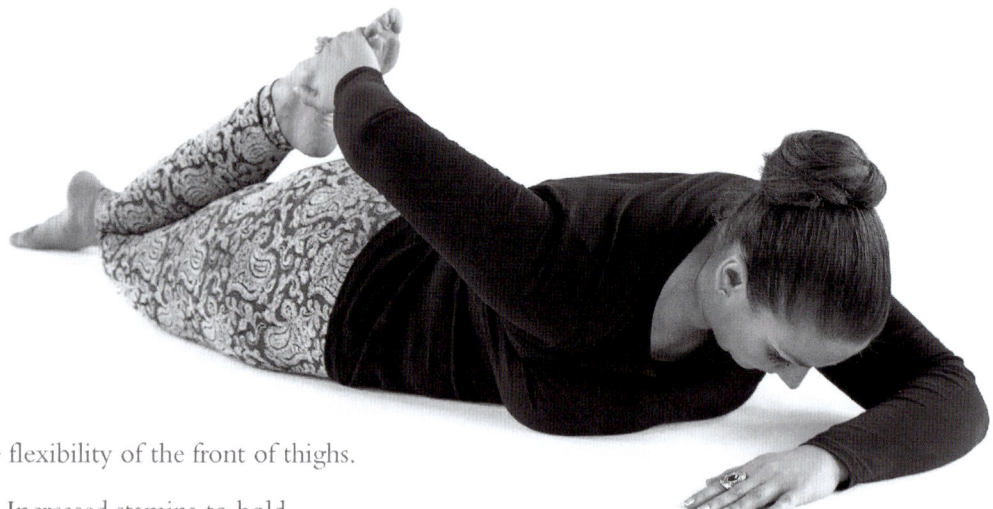

Purpose: To increase flexibility of the front of thighs.

Bedroom Pleasure: Increased stamina to hold positions and increased ability get into positions and stay for full satisfaction.

Repetitions: Hold 10-30 seconds, 1-2 sets.

1. Lying on your front, legs extended, neutral spine.

2. Keep the belly button pulled into the spine, bend the right knee, draw the heel to the booty and hold the heel, foot or trousers.

3. To increase the stretch gently press the hip into the mat or even lift the knee an inch or two off the mat and hold, always being aware of your breathing.

4. You can do a double leg front of thigh release, ensure the lower back does not become over active. Bring both heels to the booty and hold, feel the lengthening.

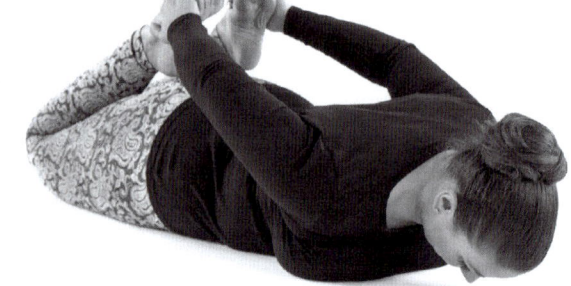

Checkpoints

- *Use the breathing to increase control and focus.*
- *Watch you do not drop through the lower back, draw the belly button in and hips tucked under.*

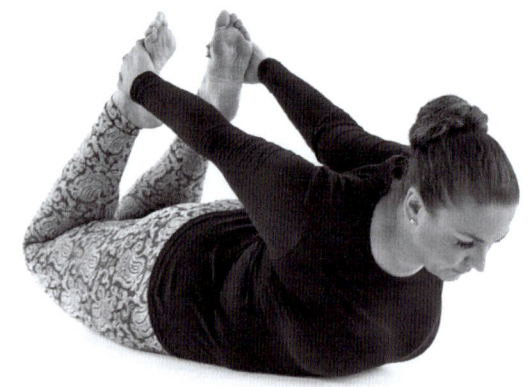

Lift & Release

The Lift & Release will gently ease muscles and relax your body and mind.

Purpose: To release and relax.

Bedroom Pleasure: Be in the moment, allowing your body and mind to connect.

Repetitions: Hold 10-30 seconds, 1-2 sets.

1. Lying on your front, allow your hands to rest under your chin, or place your forehead on your heads to ensure neutral spine.

2. Place your forearms by your sides, elbows under the shoulders. Press through the forearms lifting the upper body off the floor and hold.

3. As an option place your hands under your shoulders and extend the arms, a deeper stretch.

Smile. It lights up your face. It triggers happiness in your brain.

Checkpoints

- *Use the breathing to increase control and focus.*
- *Watch you do not drop through the lower back, draw the belly button in and hips tucked under.*

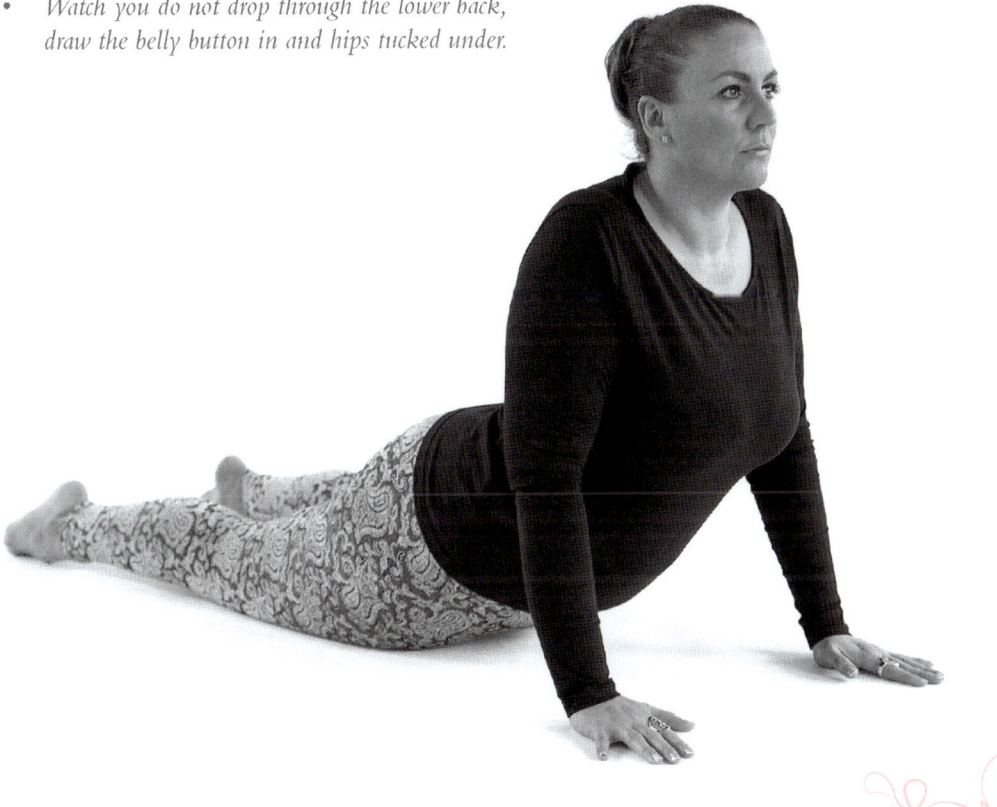

On Your Back – Hug & Release

A great stretch for your back; releasing tightness, give yourself time to tune into your body.

Purpose: To stretch and release your back.

Bedroom Pleasure: This position can transfer straight to the bedroom. Let your partner slide in.

Repetitions: Hold for up to 10 – 15 seconds, repeat 1-2 times.

1. Lying on your back bring your knees into your chest. Hold gently onto your knees or hold at the back of you thighs.

2. For a deeper stretch reach and hold your heels, really add some resistance by hugging tight, curling through the body and then release, repeat for a number of repetitions.

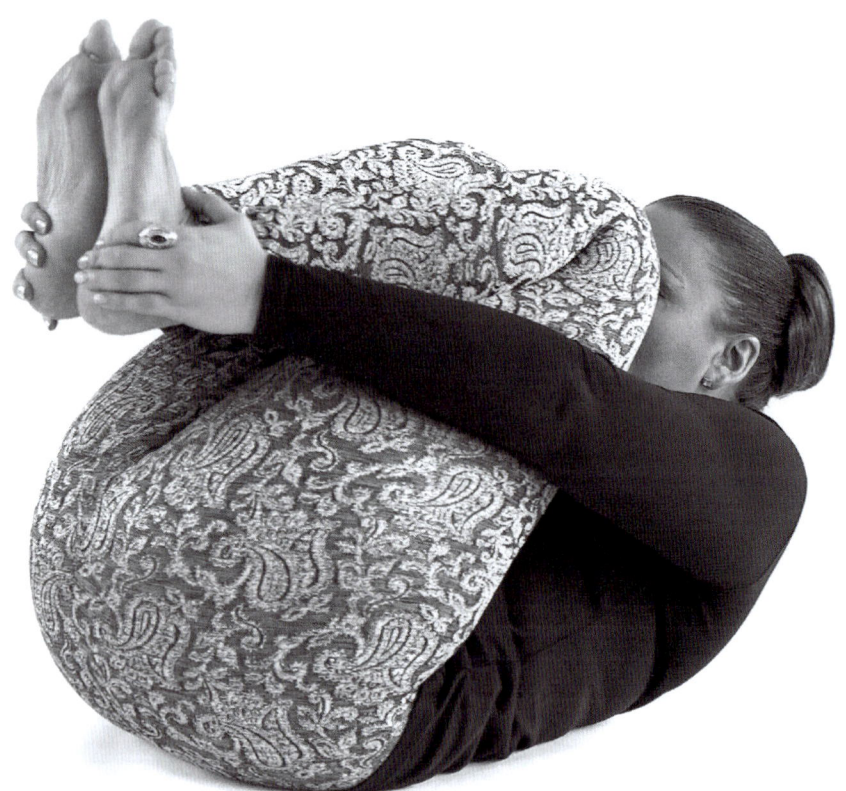

Checkpoints

- *Let the head and shoulders relax into the mat.*
- *Remember the breathing, it is tempting to want to hold the breath.*

Full Body Lengthening

A great stretch for your whole body, releasing tightness and relaxing in the moment.

Purpose: To stretch and release your whole body.

Bedroom Pleasure: Teaches you to truly relax and be in the moment.

Repetitions: Hold for up to 20-30 seconds, repeat 1-2 times.

1. Lying on your back fully extended your arms over your head and lengthen through the legs.

Checkpoints

- *Let the head and shoulders relax into the mat.*
- *Remember the breathing, it is tempting to want to hold your breath.*
- *You can focus on extending one side of the body before switching to the other side.*

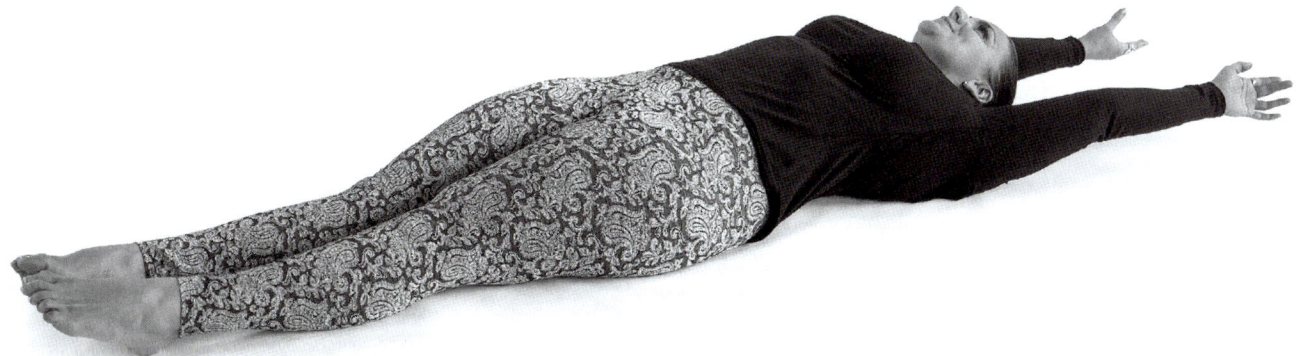

To ensure complete health and well being, ensure you monitor stress. Find something that helps you relieve it. Stay positive, love hard, laugh lots and enjoy life.

Leg Over Stretch

A great stretch for your booty; really getting in deep! Will release tightness from your booty but also the lower back. A stretch you can perform daily and truly enjoy.

Purpose: To stretch and release your booty.

Bedroom Pleasure: This stretch is a sexual position, let your partner come in from behind.

Repetitions: Hold for up to 20-30 seconds, repeat 1-2 times.

1. Lying on your back, legs extended arms soft by your sides. Neutral spine, head, shoulders and lower back relaxed into the mat.

2. Bring your right knee to the chest, gently hold over the top or come underneath the thigh, keeping the left leg long.

3. Keeping the head and shoulders to the floor take a deep breath in and as you breathe out take the knee across the body over to the left side until you feel the stretch. You will see in the photo below a leg extension, this is more advanced and gradually build up to holding this position as an option.

4. If you feel tightness in the top of the right thigh, gently lower the knee an inch or two and see if this releases to allow a deeper stretch.

5. Repeat on the other side.

Checkpoints

- *Let the head and shoulders relax into the mat. You may find yourself wanting to roll as the knee passes the midline. Fix the shoulders to the floor and rotate through the trunk.*

- *Avoid tension through the neck.*

- *Remember the breathing, it is tempting to want to hold the breath.*

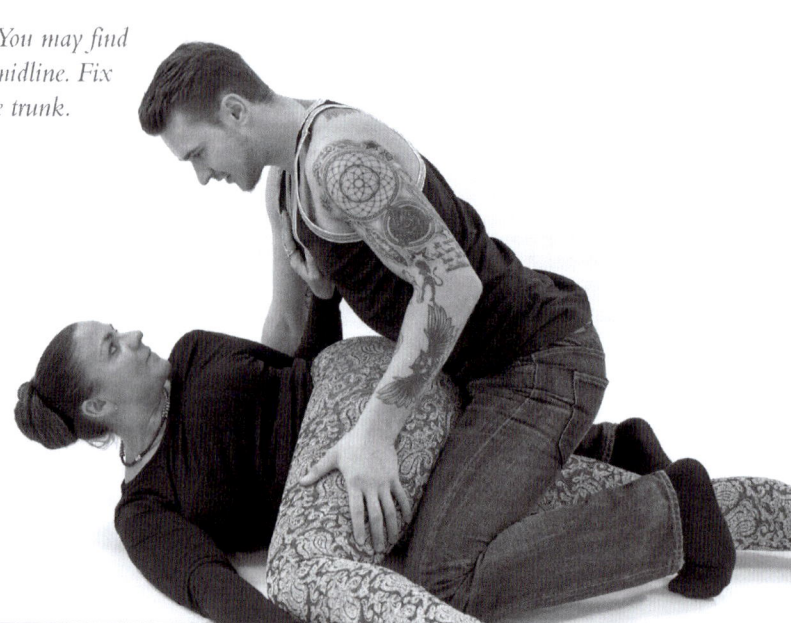

Outer Thigh

Another variation of a stretch for your booty, but this movement will also open the hip joint as well, when the lower body is mobile and flexible this means you can turn, twist and tighten your body into positions driving your partner wild……

Purpose: To stretch and release your booty.

Bedroom Pleasure: Encourage mobile hips resulting in enhanced play.

Repetitions: Hold for up to 20-30 seconds, repeat 1-2 times.

1. Lying on your back, legs extended arms soft by your sides. Neutral spine, head, shoulders and lower back relaxed into the mat.

2. Bend both knees, bring your right foot onto your left knee and open the hip. Relax into the position keeping the spine in neutral.

3. To increase the stretch, feed your hands either side of your left thigh and lift the leg off the floor keeping the head and shoulders down.

4. Repeat on the other side.

Checkpoints

- *Let the head and shoulders relax into the mat. Avoid tension through the neck.*
- *Remember the breathing, it is tempting to want to hold the breath.*
- *Keep the knee open as far as possible to add mobility to the hip.*

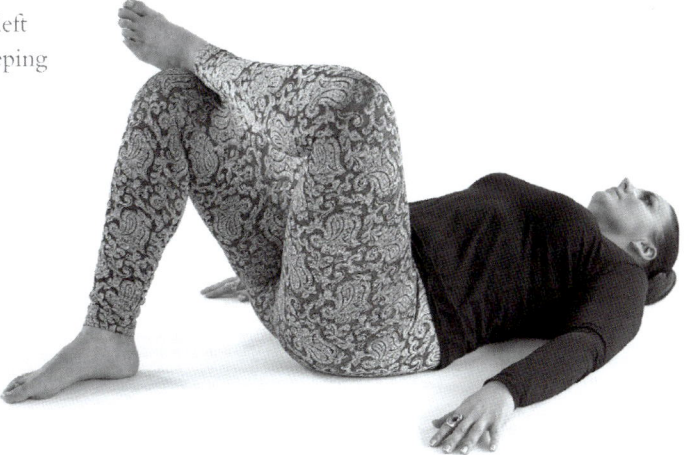

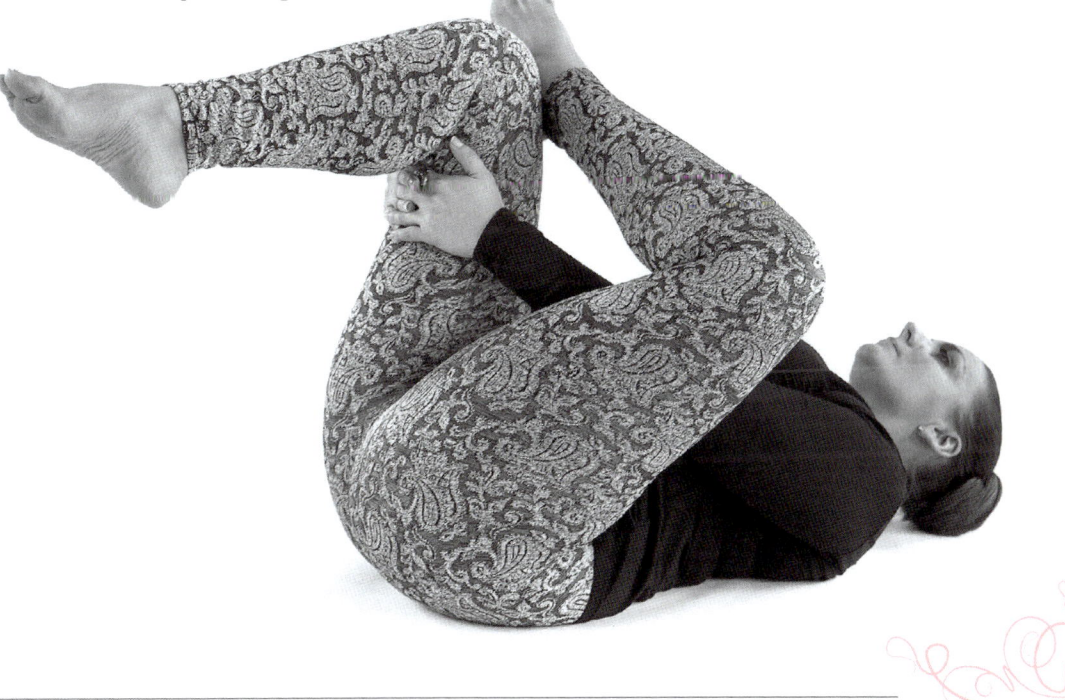

Full Leg Lengthening

A deep stretch for the back of the leg, particularly the thigh and behind the knee; release at its greatest! Many suffer tightness in the back of thighs and when we attempt sexual positions from the Karma Sutra; tight thighs will hinder our performance and limit our pleasure.

Purpose: To stretch and increase flexibility of the back of thighs.

Bedroom Pleasure: Increased flexibility means legs can be held in all positions and the va va voom increases.

Repetitions: Hold for up to 20-30 seconds, repeat 1-2 times.

1. Lying on your back, legs extended arms soft by your sides. Neutral spine, head, shoulders and lower back relaxed into the mat.

2. You have the optional to bend the knees if this supports the lower back or keep the legs resting on the mat.

3. Extend the right leg to the ceiling. Keep the leg as straight as you comfortably can, foot relaxed. Hold the leg at the back of the thigh, on the calf or right by the ankle (depending on flexibility). Always ensure you can breathe naturally throughout. You should feel the stretch but no excessive shaking.

4. There is the option for a double leg full lengthening. Deeper more intense. Sign up for more ideas and routines; visit www.pilatesforbettersex.com.

5. Repeat on the other side.

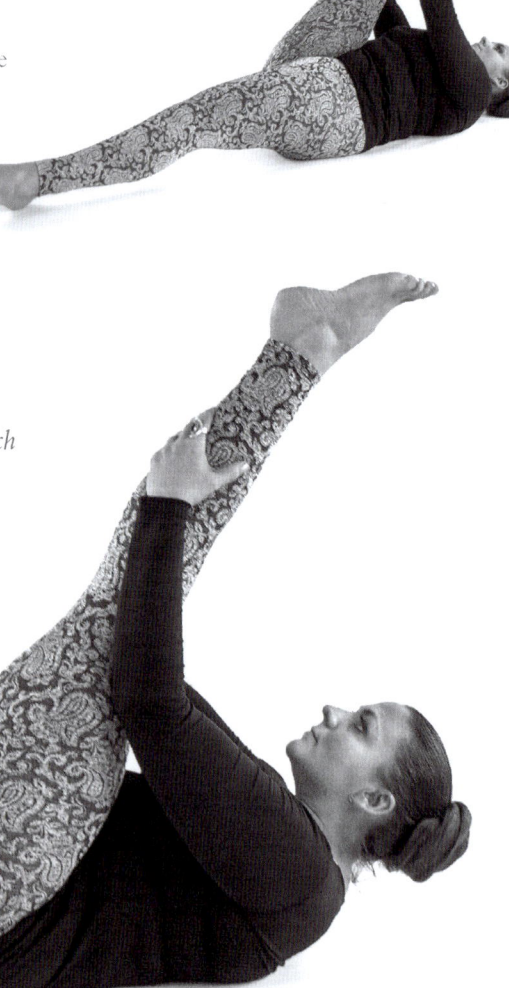

Checkpoints

- *Let the head and shoulders relax into the mat. Avoid tension through the neck. Though some women prefer to resist into the stretch you are welcome to lift the head and shoulder whilst gently adding some resistance to the leg and release for a few repetitions.*

- *Remember the breathing, it is tempting to want to hold the breath.*

Let It Flow

Visit **www.pilatesforbettersex.com** for more ideas on routines for all levels.

Curl & Release	71
Sit Back And Hold	72
Front Of Thigh	74
Lift & Release	75
Shoulder Release	70
Inner Thigh	73
Full Body Lengthening	77
Hug & Release	76

Chapter 6

Positions of Pleasure

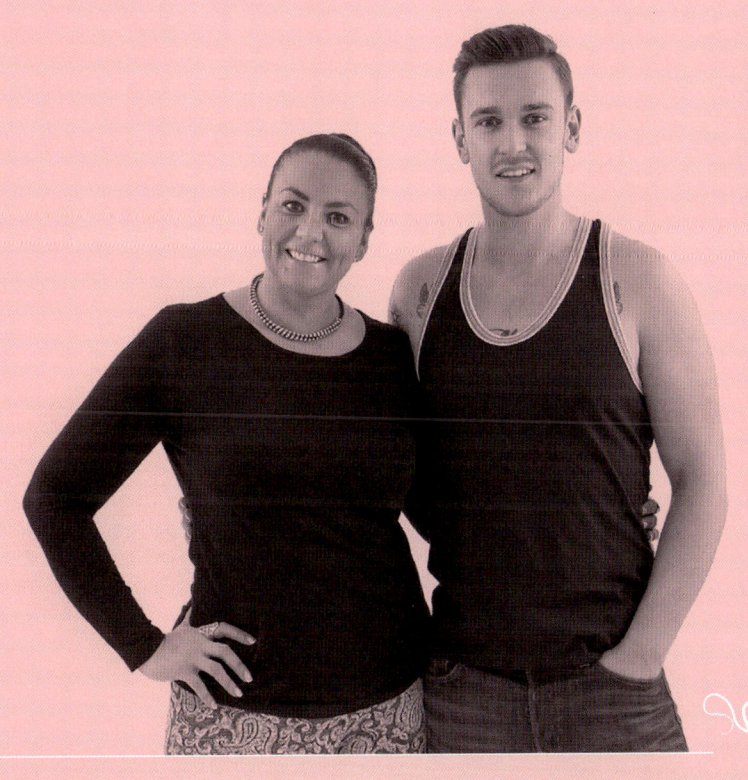

Positions of Pleasure

Take it Slow – Time for foreplay

Now you have the moves, if you want more pleasure please sign up at www.pilatesforbettersex.com. Take the positions below and really turn the heat up in the bedroom.

Treasure

Remember first dating your partner? Would you wear sexy underwear in the hopes you would make love? Did you experiment with seduction and sexual techniques? You treasured your new love. In other words, you made an effort. Over time, many often sexually neglect each other. If so, mindful sex can reconnect and heal. Whatever the past, begin again, right where you are. Treasure your love, take time to remember the early days, honour their mind, their heart and their body. See them through fresh eyes and trace their skin with your fingertips, your lips and your mouth.

Tantalise

Start by recreating the delicious anticipation you used to feel about connecting sexually with your partner. Create an event. Prepare to tantalise all of your lover's senses—perhaps lighting candles, playing music and laying out warm scented massage oils, chocolate, berries and bubbles. Think and take time for foreplay, be mindful. Carefully plan for passion and then let go into the present moment, embrace and enjoy.

Tune In

Begin by facing each other and gazing deeply into each other's eyes. It is most powerful to focus on one eye; this keeps you intimately exposed (some people look back and forth between the two eyes to reduce the intensity...but that's cheating). Next, synchronise your breathing – breathe in together, exhale together. Then try breath exchange – you inhale when they exhale, you exhale when they inhale, as though you are breathing each other in and out. Feel the distractions settle and the worries melt away. Really look, really see, and allow yourself to be seen. Gently draw in close and connect, be connected.

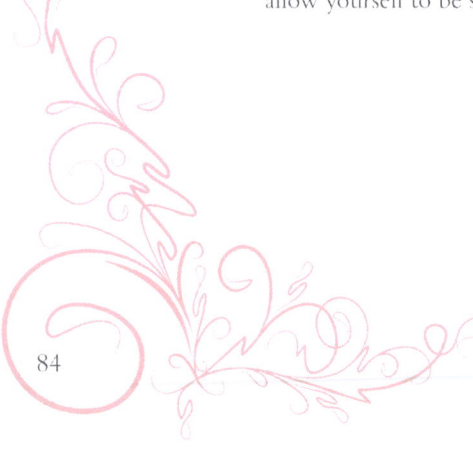

Tease

Begin slowly and mindfully undressing each other. Take turns. Slowly, ever so slowly, tease and arouse your lover's whole body, eventually caressing their most sensitive parts. Invite them to sigh or moan, blending your touch with their sounds. Bring them to the edge of orgasm, then back. Repeat. Reverse roles. Give, receive, exchange, and explore. See if you can drive each other wild with anticipation for what comes next.

Transform

With mindful sex, excitement and pleasure are just the beginning. The focus is on slowing down, staying in the moment, and allowing profound sexual and emotional merging. Instead of swooning away from your partner and into your own orgasm, you cultivate and sustain the sexual ecstasy. You then share the energy of your orgasm. To practice this, stay connected with your lover's eyes and breathe as you make love and approach orgasm. Just before the peak, focus on the impending waves of pleasure. As the orgasm waves begin to move through your lower body, stay present.

Allow

Allow everything else to fall away except for your eye contact, your breathing, and your beating hearts.

Here are some of my all time favourites, now remember don't just 'do it' take the moment, be in the moment, feel the moment.

Mission to the Moon

Despite being one of the most passive positions for a woman, with your man on top can still provide one amazing experience; if you connect. Connect with your partners thrusting, feel the energy, flow together, think of your pelvic peeling & the booty brace, accentuate riding towards him to really allow your pelvic muscles to grip his shaft. He will love being in control but it drives a man wild to feel you being pleasured, let your body talk to him.

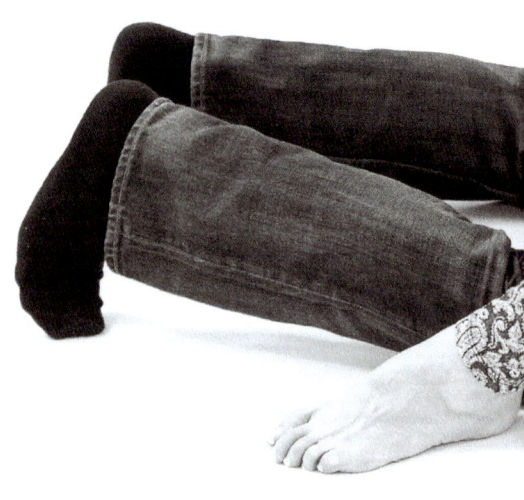

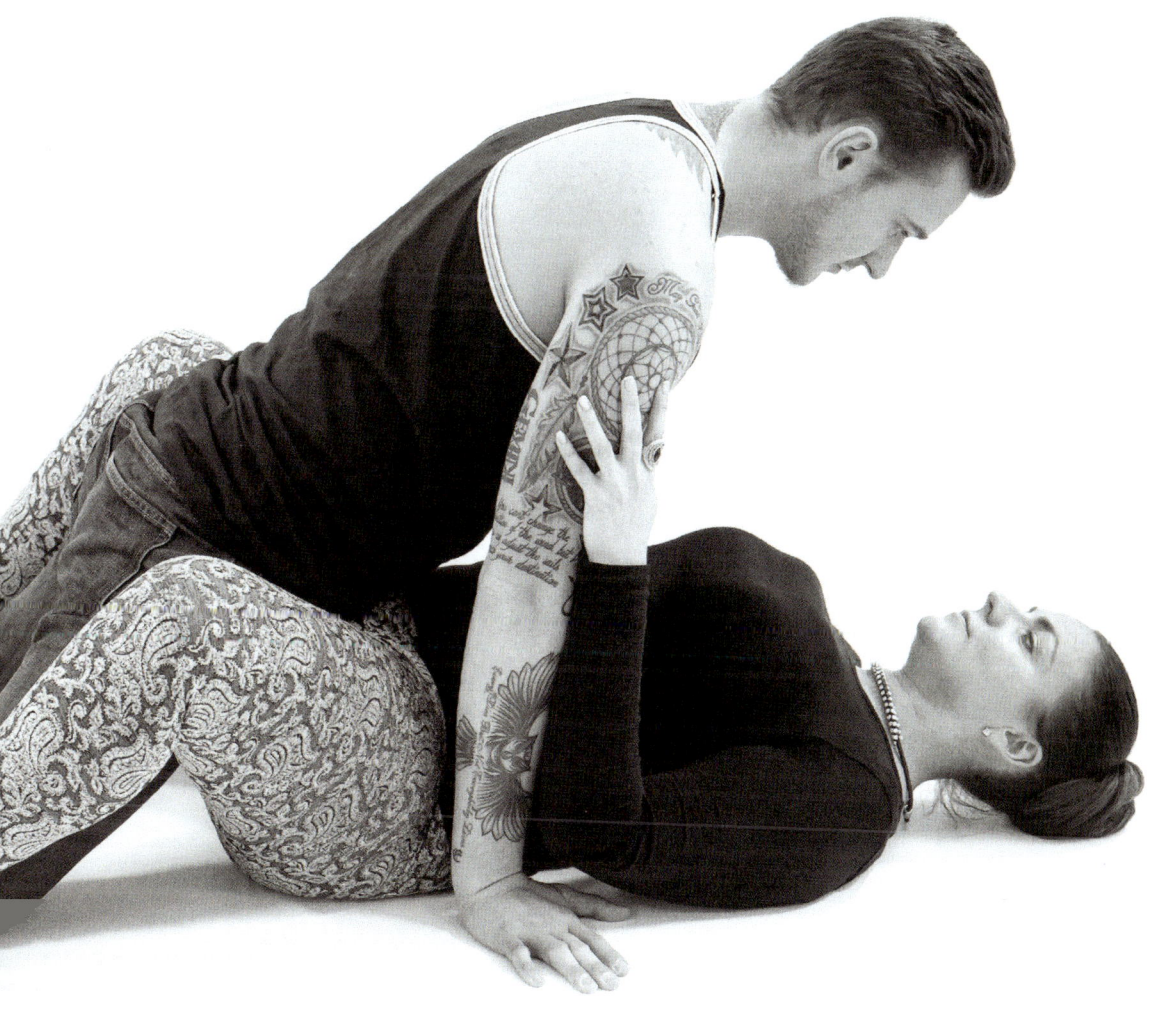

Booty from Behind

Penetration from behind will engage your core as you have to stabilise. You need good upper and lower body strength to perform this position for time, but to maximise the experience, mobilise the spine, tilt those hips, open up the pelvis, accentuate your booty and explore the following options; on all fours, leaning over the bed and up against a wall, try them all.

Pilates for Better Sex

The Rider

Your legs are straddled on the bed or floor and you will need to engage your booty and core. Then much like riding a horse, flex and relax your lower core and pelvic muscles.

To truly intensify, slightly tilt those mobilised hips, gently press your clitoris into his groin and as you move, embrace the penetration and stimulation. Double pleasure. Also, don't forget reverse rider! If he is a booty man, reverse rider will drive him wild.

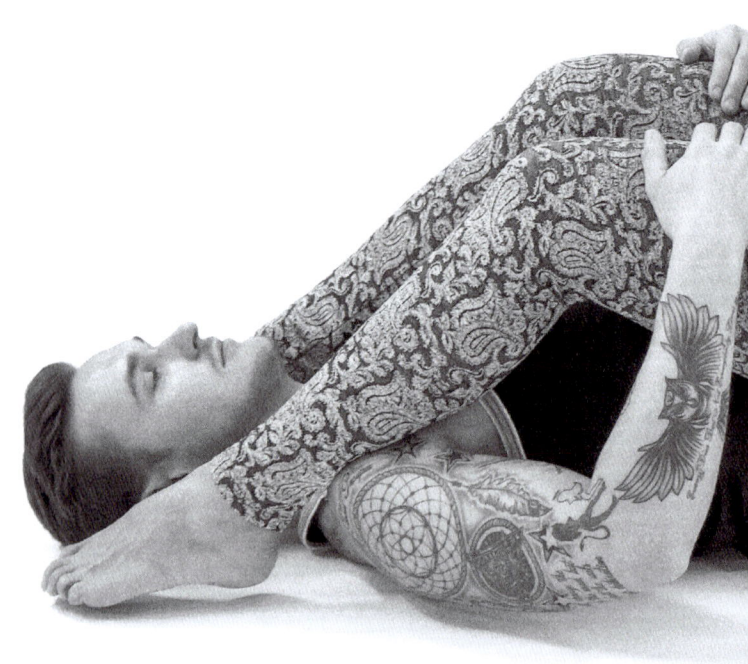

Pilates for Better Sex

Flamingo

Standing is one of the more challenging positions, you do need lower body strength and to truly maximise the experience, be able to hold the position and work those pelvic muscles at the same time. Trust in your partner to support some of your weight or use a wall. Stand on one leg and tilt your hips, if your partner slightly lifts your booty, this will allow for a deeper thrust. As with any of these positions, connecting together will intensify the sexual pleasure, let your bodies tune in together and the sweet music will be felt and heard.

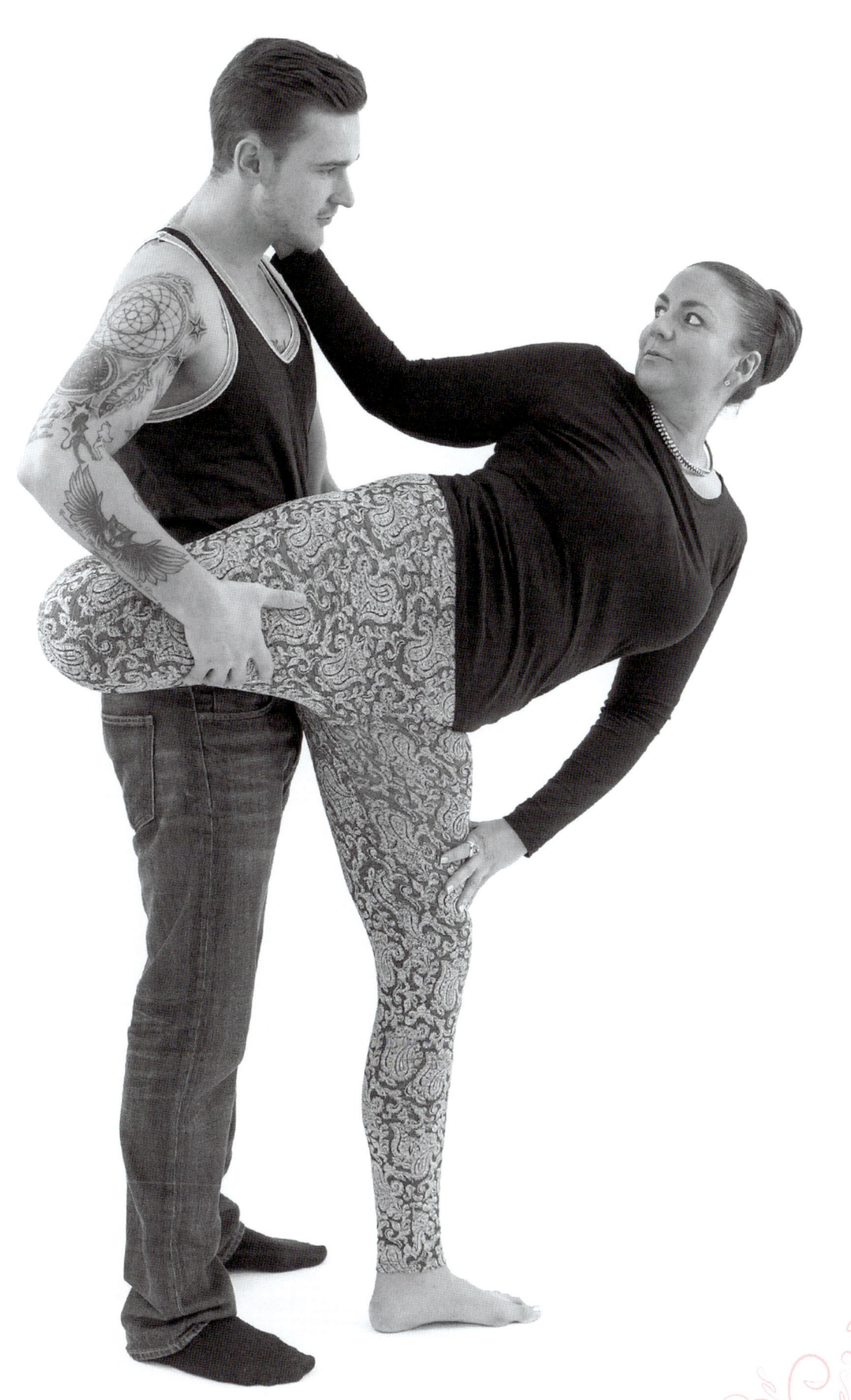

Side Lie Loving

The traditional spoon, with similar benefits to the Booty from Behind, this really allows you to get intimate and close, to be in each others energy. The stability provided from the floor or the bed means you can truly engage your pelvic floor, allow your partner to glide deep, slow, hard and fast. Explore tender kisses, stroking and touching. Face to face side lie, why not tilt your hips, lift one leg and gently rock forward and back and take control of the movement, engage the core, use your flexibility and muscle control and enjoy!

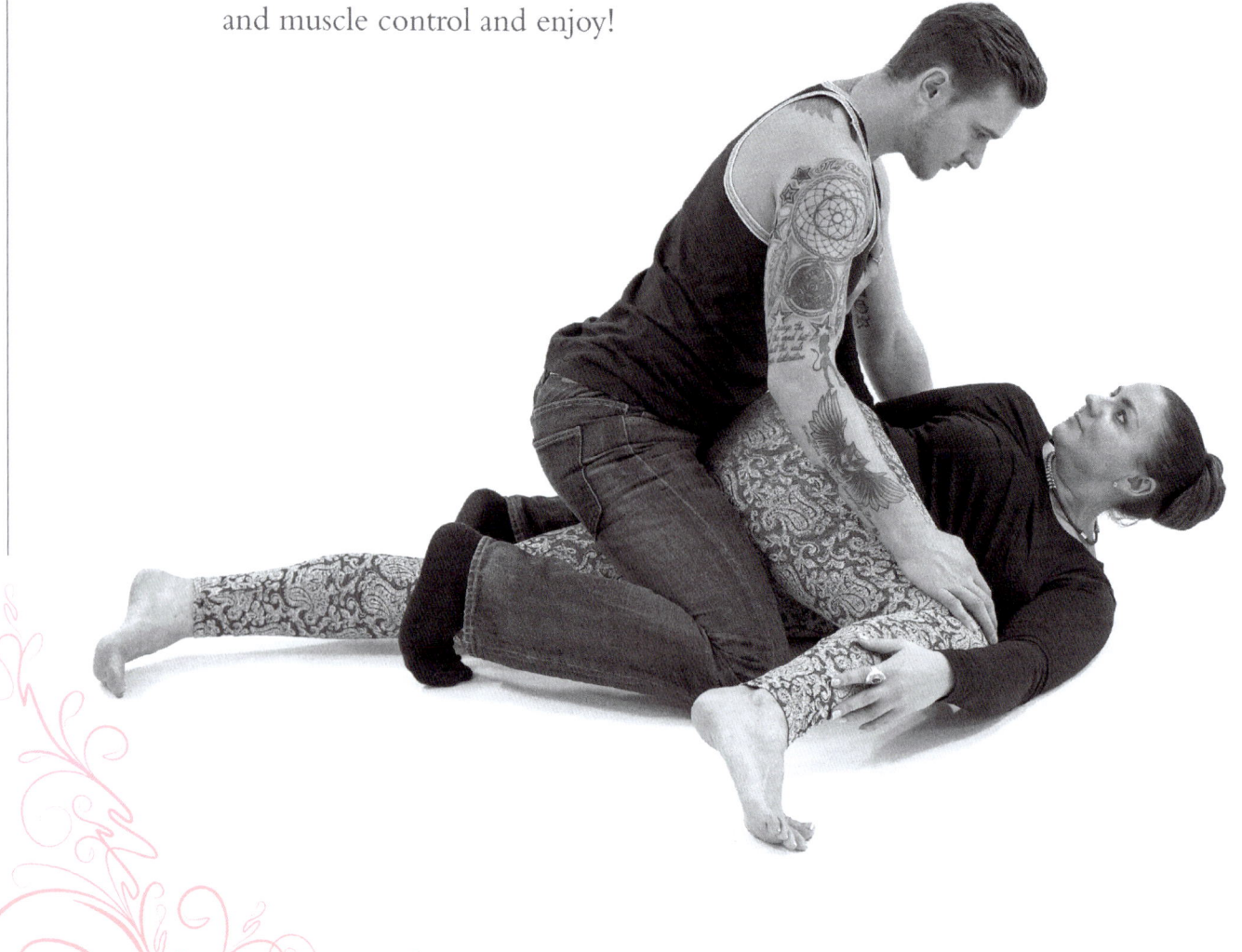

Printed in Great Britain
by Amazon